DR SADJA GREENWOOD lives and works in San Francisco, California, where she is well-known for her work on women's health programmes.

She is Medical Director of a local health centre and an Assistant Professor at the University of California Medical Center, San Francisco. She is also active in many well women clinics in the San Francisco area.

Dr Greenwood, a mother of two grown-up sons, describes herself as 'looking for the truths about life and the joy in every day'.

MENOPAUSE
THE NATURAL WAY

DR SADJA GREENWOOD

ILLUSTRATED BY SUSAN HELLARD

An OPTIMA book

© 1984, 1987 by Sadja Greenwood
A previous edition of this book was published by
Volcano Press, Inc in 1984.
This edition published by arrangement with
Volcano Press, Inc, San Francisco, California, USA.
© 1987 British edition Macdonald & Co (Publishers) Ltd

First published in Great Britain in 1987
by Optima, a division of Macdonald & Co (Publishers) Ltd
Reprinted 1990

A member of Maxwell Macmillan Pergamon Publishing Corporation

British Library Cataloguing in Publication Data
Greenwood, Sadja
    Menopause the natural way. –2nd. ed.
    1. Women. Menopause
    I. Title
    612.665

    ISBN 0-356-19692-5

Macdonald & Co (Publishers) Ltd
Orbit House
1 New Fetter Lane
London EC4A 1AR

Photoset by ⫝̸ Tek Art Limited, Croydon, Surrey
Printed in Great Britain by
BPCC Hazell Books
Aylesbury, Bucks, England
Member of BPCC Ltd.

CONTENTS

1. FACTS, FALLACIES, AND NEW POSSIBILITIES   9

2. HOWS AND WHYS OF MENSTRUAL BLEEDING   15
   Hormonal imbalance and irregular ovulation   17
   Uterine fibroids   21
   Cancer or overgrowth of the uterine lining   24
   Cancer of the cervix   25
   Positive aspects of the menopause   26

3. THE OVARIES – HIDDEN SOURCES OF WELL-BEING   27
   The menopause with ovaries but no uterus   30

4. HOT FLUSHES AND HOW TO SURVIVE THEM   31
   What causes hot flushes   33
   What's behind hot flushes?   34
   Living with hot flushes   35
   Treatment for hot flushes   36

5. SEX IN THE SECOND HALF OF LIFE   38
   Vaginal dryness and lovemaking   39
   Kegel's exercises   41
   Irritation, incontinence, and infection   43
   Birth control   43
   Hysterectomy and sexuality   43

6. YOUR LOOKS IN THE MENOPAUSAL YEARS   46
   Weight gain   47
   Skin changes   48
   Loss of flexibility   50
   Sex appeal   50

7. KEEPING YOUR BONES STRONG   52
    The biology of osteoporosis   52
    Who's at risk?   54
    Oestrogen and osteoporosis   62

8. HORMONES AND EMOTIONAL IMBALANCE   65
    Cultural factors   66
    Hormonal factors   69

9. WHEN PERIODS STOP BEFORE FORTY   73
    Conditions that are not premature menopause   74
    What is premature menopause?   74
    Pregnancy and premature menopause   75
    Early menopause from surgery   75
    Replacement hormones   76

10. HORMONE REPLACEMENT THERAPY (HRT)   78
    A little history   79
    Oestrogen – types and methods of use   81
    Use of a progestogen with oestrogen   82
    Reasons for taking post-menopausal oestrogens   84
    What HRT won't do   87
    Reasons for not taking post-menopausal oestrogens   87
    Controversies over HRT   89

11. SHOULD YOU HAVE HRT?   93
    The decision to use HRT – a personal rating scale   94
    Advantages of HRT   95
    Disadvantages of HRT   98

12. POST-MENOPAUSAL ZEST   102
    Beliefs about ageing   103
    Staying connected to the world around you   106

13. RELAXATION – CALMING DOWN AND LETTING GO   109
    Relaxation techniques   112

14. EXERCISE IN MIDLIFE   115
     Heart disease   115
     Osteoporosis   118
     Weight control   119
     Appearance   120
     Depression, moods, and sleep   120
     How to start exercising   120

15. DIET AND THE MENOPAUSE   123
     Whole grains   123
     Beans   125
     Vegetables   125
     Fruits   127
     Meat, poultry, and fish   128
     Milk, yogurt, and cheese   129
     Eggs   130
     Fats   131
     Sugar   132
     Salt   134
     Alcohol   135
     Caffeine   138
     Making changes in your diet   140

16. VITAMIN AND MINERAL SUPPLEMENTS   141
     Calcium   142
     Multivitamins   143

17. GIVING UP SMOKING   145

18. HEALTHCARE   148

19. SUMMING IT ALL UP!   151

     USEFUL ADDRESSES   154

     INDEX   158

1.
FACTS, FALLACIES, AND NEW POSSIBILITIES

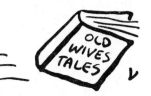

Cecilia walked rapidly into my office and pulled out her notes. 'Look at this record of my periods,' she said with despair. 'I'm probably going through the menopause at 42. It's ironic that I'll fall apart at a time when I've finally found the right job and a good relationship.' After listening to Cecilia and examining her, I explained to her that her frequent heavy periods were not a sign of the menopause, but might be related to a small fibroid tumour on her uterus, or to her increasing use of alcohol to calm herself after long hours of exacting work. I found that she considered the menopause to be a tragic time in life because of vivid memories of her mother's problems after having a hysterectomy at the age of 40. Her mother's regrets over this surgical menopause had greatly influenced Cecilia's early life.

Later in the same day Paula was telling me about her intense feelings of irritability and depression before her periods. 'Is this what it's like to go through the menopause?' she asked. 'If so, I'm really dreading it.'

Neither of these women was actually going through the menopause, but both showed me that they needed information and a more positive view about this natural transition between the years of fertility and the second half of life. Negative messages about the menopause abound in our culture – in cartoons, old wives' tales, and even medical texts. Fear and dread of the 'change of life' are easy to acquire and can influence our behaviour, our beliefs, and our bodies in subtly destructive ways.

Lillian, a Chinese woman of 50, viewed her menopause more positively. Her periods had stopped in her late forties. Lillian said, 'Getting rid of my periods was such a relief to me. I feel very balanced now. I took up Tai Chi about ten years ago because I was getting sluggish, and that has made a big difference in my life. I do it every morning before work.' Listening to Lillian made me reflect that she came from a culture with more respect for ageing. She had also found a daily exercise that increased her strength and her feelings of inner harmony. Her menopause had been a smooth transition.

As a doctor, I am always gathering information about the way

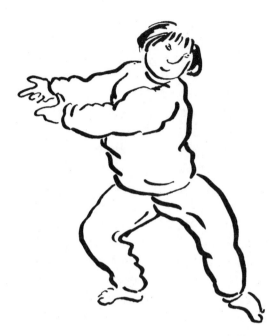

people lead their daily lives and the way they feel about themselves. I have found that women who enter the menopause viewing it as a natural process or transition have an easier time than those who view it as a crisis. Women who exercise daily, eat healthy food, and work on achieving emotional balance usually manage to avoid many of the ills of midlife. Moreover, adopting such practices can cure many problems more reliably than drugs or surgery. A skilful doctor can help patients decide when counselling and lifestyle changes are sufficient, or when medicine or life saving technology is needed.

In recent years I have conducted a special clinic for midlife women and have taken part in numerous discussion groups on the menopause. I have been impressed by the help that women can give to each other in open discussions, and by the power of accurate, non-threatening information.

An open discussion and explanation of the menopause helped Claudia to see her own future as different from her mother's. 'You

11

mean I don't have to go crazy in the menopause?' Claudia laughed at herself as she asked this question, but there was an edge of fear in her voice. 'Whenever I think of my mother and her depressions I get really worried.' When she analyzed it, Claudia wasn't so sure that her mother was more depressed in the menopause than she had been years earlier or later. However, she had heard other relatives blame her mother's condition on 'the change of life' and had accepted this explanation. Years later, as she approached the menopause herself, she found that she had an irrational dread of reliving her mother's example.

What does happen in the menopause? Strictly speaking, the word menopause refers only to the final menstrual period. In common usage, however, it designates a transitional time from a few years before the last period to a year after it. As hormone output from the ovaries declines, menstrual periods become irregular and then disappear. Symptoms such as hot flushes, night sweats, and vaginal dryness are experienced at this time by four out of five women. The menopause usually occurs between 48 and 52, but it often happens earlier and occasionally later.

We don't know why the menopause occurs in human beings but not in animals. Anthropologists have suggested that the menopause has benefited our species during evolution, by releasing women from the stresses and dangers of childbearing to bring up any late-born children and transmit cultural knowledge. They also point out that the menopausal transition is viewed very differently from one society to another. In Western culture, with its strong emphasis on female youth and beauty, the menopause is seen as a time of decline and loss of status for women. It is viewed as a medical event – even a disease process – which requires treatment and careful medical follow-up. Other societies see the menopause very differently. Among many non-Western groups, the older woman enjoys increased status in the family and greater freedom in society at large. The menopause and the cessation of childbearing become positive events in a woman's life, and physical symptoms are given less attention.

Since the 1960s, profound changes have occurred in women's

perceptions of their rights and roles in our society. Women are more active in every phase of community life, and more aware of their own needs and directions. This development has been linked to momentous changes in women's health care, including the ability to choose when or whether to have children, and a driving need on the part of many women to understand their bodies and participate in decisions about their own health or illness. Today, as millions of women reach their forties and fifties they are seeking new approaches to the menopause.

Belle looked like she had a lot to say, and I listened intently to her story. 'At first the menopause was very difficult for me. I was waking up at night with hot flushes and couldn't get back to sleep. I felt very self-conscious at work whenever I had one. My daughter was driving me crazy, which didn't help. My doctor said I should take oestrogen pills, but they made my breasts extremely sore and gave me a funny feeling in my head. Then a friend of mine at work started taking me to her yoga class. That really turned things around for me. I suppose I learned how to relax for the first time in my life. My body felt better, I stopped the oestrogen and started taking vitamins. The hot flushes still come but they don't bother me any more. I've learned so much in that class that I think I feel healthier than when I was 30.' Belle did a yoga posture to show me how supple she had become. I was also impressed that her blood pressure was low and her heart rate slow and even.

Women like Belle want to replace the negative stereotypes of the menopausal woman with a more positive outlook. This viewpoint will flourish as women learn more about how to live through the changes of middle age with maximum health and equanimity.

I have two major aims in this book – to provide as much information as possible on how to promote good health and avoid illness in the second half of life, and to discuss interesting and controversial questions about the menopause – such as why bleeding is irregular and hot flushes occur, how to deal with vaginal soreness, how to make an informed decision about oestrogen use (hormone replacement therapy), and how to avoid brittle bones (osteoporosis).

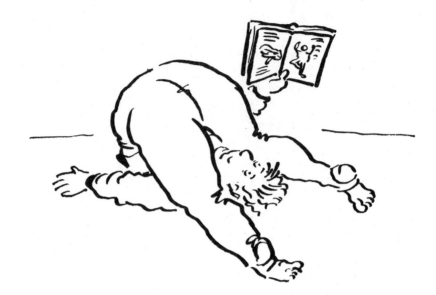

Margaret Mead, the well-known anthropologist, spoke about 'post-menopausal zest'. I've seen women who have post-menopausal zest and those who don't, and those who find it after a long process of self-exploration and self-healing. Perhaps I can show you some short cuts along the way.

2.
HOWS AND WHYS OF MENSTRUAL BLEEDING

One month I can hardly get out of the house because of the bleeding I'm having, and the next month there's almost nothing. I never know what to expect these days.

My periods are getting closer together and sometimes they are really heavy. Is that normal at 48?

Last month my period didn't come at all. I started waking up at night feeling really hot, and I couldn't get back to sleep. Then I had another period and everything is back to normal.

My husband died when I was 49. It was a terrible time. I never had another period after his death, but I never had any menopausal symptoms either.

All these and many other patterns can occur in the menopause. Let's review what is known about menstruation and its somewhat erratic behaviour at this time of life. The uterus is a pear-shaped organ that develops a lining of cells and blood vessels every month in the fertile years. A menstrual period occurs when the uterus sheds this lining. This happens at regular intervals to most women under 45.

Each month the ovaries produce the hormones oestrogen and progesterone in a predictable pattern. Oestrogen is produced in the first half of the cycle in increasing amounts, causing a thick lining to grow in the uterus. At mid-cycle one ovary produces a mature egg cell, or ovum, which travels down a narrow tube into the uterus. This event is called ovulation, and marks the time when pregnancy can occur. After ovulation, in the two weeks before the next menstrual period, the ovary produces progesterone as well as oestrogen. This causes the uterine lining to prepare for pregnancy by secreting special fluids and stabilizing the growth of the lining cells. When pregnancy does not occur, the ovaries stop their hormone production, oestrogen and progesterone levels decrease rapidly, and the uterine lining loses its hormonal support and begins to break down. This lining is shed during the menstrual period, so the body can prepare for next month's egg cell. This is the monthly rhythm of women in their fertile years.

As women reach their mid-forties, on the average, ovulation becomes less regular, and hormonal output may vary. Many women notice their periods are closer together at this time. The amount of bleeding may be lighter than before, but occasionally it is very heavy. Sometimes, when ovulation does not occur, a period is skipped. Failure to ovulate can also cause prolonged 'spotting' and erratic bleeding, since the ovaries do not secrete progesterone until ovulation occurs. In the absence of progesterone, oestrogen levels tend to rise and fall and the lining is shed very irregularly. After a time of such erratic bleeding, ovulation may recur and normal periods are resumed.

Around the age of 50, menstrual periods will generally get further apart and lighter, and then stop entirely. Some women experience this final pause before 50, some after. Very few women still menstruate at the age of 55. When a woman has had a year or two without bleeding around the age of 50, she has completed the time known as the menopause, and should sail smoothly into a new phase of middle life.

Many variations of bleeding patterns can occur as women enter the menopause. Some are normal, but others may indicate problems. It's typical for periods to be closer together at first, with heavier bleeding from time to time. Timing may be unpredictable. Later on, periods become scantier in flow and further apart. Occasionally there is just spotting for a month or two. Some women cease menstruating abruptly, after a psychological shock or after stopping the birth control pill in their forties.

The bleeding pattern most troublesome to women and worrying to doctors is repeated very heavy bleeding, especially if it is irregular. This can cause discomfort and anaemia, and may be the result of hormonal imbalance, uterine fibroids (benign tumours on the wall of the uterus), or cancer. Let us consider these factors and their treatment one by one.

HORMONAL IMBALANCE AND IRREGULAR OVULATION

By far the most common cause of irregular heavy bleeding among women in their late forties is lack of ovulation and a resultant hormonal imbalance. When this situation occurs the cause is usually the production of too much oestrogen and too little progesterone. There are various reasons for the problem, including the natural process of ageing. However, frequently factors such as excessive stress can make the situation worse. Let's examine how this problem is usually treated, and then look at how it can be prevented from recurring.

When bleeding is prolonged or very heavy in the menopausal years, most doctors will first advise a minor operation known as a dilatation and curettage (D and C) to stop the bleeding and rule out cancer. In this procedure the lining of the uterus is removed, by suction or a scraping technique, and then analyzed for any abnormality. It can be done under a local or general anaesthetic. Usually cancer is not found, and everyone is greatly relieved. However, after a D and C the uterine lining will grow back, and irregular bleeding may recur.

At this point the woman is often advised to take a hormone supplement called a progestogen – similar to progesterone. Since progesterone, secreted by the ovary after ovulation, stabilizes the growth of the uterine lining, the use of a progestogen usually stops irregular bleeding. The body responds as if ovulation had occurred. The progestogen is taken for one or two weeks and when it is stopped, bleeding will recur, usually lasting less than a week, like a normal period. In many cases the irregular bleeding will not return in the next cycle. If it does, the progestogen can be taken again. Occasionally the use of a progestogen may cause feelings of tiredness, increased appetite, and other symptoms, but there are seldom serious side effects.

Since many women would prefer to prevent such problems rather than take medicines when they occur, let's examine some natural remedies that make hormone imbalance and abnormal bleeding less likely:

Reduce Emotional Upsets: Emotional upset can have a profound effect on the reproductive system, causing little or no bleeding in some women and extensive or prolonged bleeding in others. Why is this so? In our long evolutionary history it has been better for the human species that fewer pregnancies occur in times of great social or personal disruption, or during prolonged episodes of exertion, exhaustion, famine or fear. These protective mechanisms are still at work in our bodies. When we experience strong and prolonged negative emotions, the area in the brain that controls ovarian function may not operate well, ovulation may become irregular, and various hormonal problems can occur. Menstrual periods may stop completely or bleeding may be erratic and persistent. When the stressful situation is resolved, women often resume a more regular bleeding schedule. For older women, this will mean a smoother transition into the menopause.

How do you resolve the stress of a serious family illness, a difficult marriage, or overwhelming financial problems? Each of us must find our own way, giving ourselves time to consult our inner wisdom. Sometimes counselling is an answer, sometimes prayer or meditation, sometimes decisive action. When a start toward resolution is made, many disturbed body functions will improve.

Give Up Smoking: Smokers often have problems with abnormal bleeding. Substances in cigarette smoke, such as nicotine and carbon monoxide, enter the blood stream and are damaging to the ovaries, causing them to stop ovulating too early. Hence smokers enter the menopause earlier than non-smokers and may have a more difficult time. Cigarette smoking also causes tension, rapid pulse, and easy exhaustion. All these factors make women more susceptible to irregular bleeding.

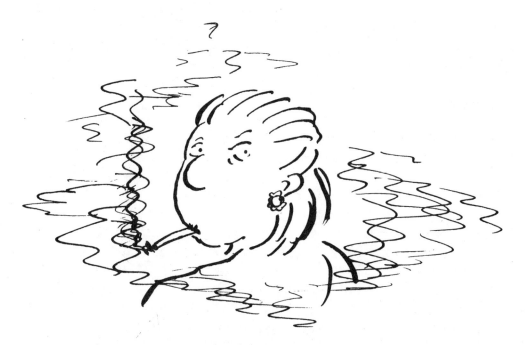

Drink Moderately: Drinking alcohol in small amounts on social occasions is a pleasure for many people. However, alcohol in large quantities has a toxic effect on many parts of the body. For example, it affects the ovaries, causing a decline in ovulation and hormone production. As a consequence, heavy drinkers often experience irregular and erratic bleeding, which usually clears up when the drinking stops.

Claire began to have extremely heavy and irregular periods at the age of 48. She worked as a waitress so she needed a lot of energy every day, but during her periods she felt exhausted. A discussion and physical examination revealed that she was very worried about money and was drinking too much. Her husband was out of work and they both drank beer all evening. They ate frozen dinners or cheese and crackers – whatever was easiest. Claire listened dubiously as I explained that alcohol, stress, and poor nutrition might be affecting her menstrual cycles. She tried taking progestogens but the problem came back whenever she stopped. Finally her husband got a new job and decided to join the Alcoholics Anonymous. Claire went to some meetings with him and also decided to give up drinking. They both began to eat a healthier diet. In about three-months Claire's periods were back to normal, and subsequently she started the menopause without further problems.

As we age we are more affected by drugs of all kinds, including alcohol, because our bodies break them down and excrete them more slowly. In the menopause it's wise to drink only small amounts (a little wine or beer on social occasions) and to give it up completely if you have bleeding problems.

Cut Down On Caffeine: We know a lot about the effects of caffeine (in coffee, tea, some cola drinks, and chocolate) on the nervous system, the heart, and the digestive system. It stimulates the brain to think more rapidly, banishes fatigue, and causes muscle tension. It stimulates the heart to beat more rapidly and forcefully, sometimes causing unpleasant feelings of pounding and skipped beats. It causes more acid secretion in the stomach, worsening the problem of ulcers.

But what does caffeine do to the woman's reproductive system? There is very little research in this area, except for recent suggestions that large amounts of coffee in pregnancy may cause birth defects. Many doctors believe excessive caffeine intake in midlife may cause constant feelings of tension and hypersensitivity to stimuli. This chronic stress can lead to disturbances in the output of hormones and menstrual irregularities. Some women find that irregular heavy menstrual bleeding reverts to normal when they stop overstimulating their nervous systems with caffeine. Frequently people who drink a lot of coffee or tea also smoke cigarettes and then use alcohol to calm their 'coffee nerves'. The woman with bleeding problems needs to become free of dependence on all these drugs to establish a more normal menstrual rhythm or a smoother transition into the menopause.

UTERINE FIBROIDS

Some women in their fertile years develop irregular enlargements or tumours on the wall of the uterus, known as fibroids (also called myomas, or fibromyomas). Fibroids are almost never cancerous. Their growth is stimulated by ovarian hormones, especially oestrogen. As a result, their growth generally diminishes in the late forties, as oestrogen levels drop, and they actually shrink after the menopause, rarely creating any further problems.

Fibroids may cause pressure on the bowel or bladder, and such heavy menstrual bleeding that the woman may become seriously anaemic, or unable to carry on her daily activities. The uterus can grow to the size of a four or five month pregnancy. For such reasons it is clear to some women that a hysterectomy (surgical removal of the uterus) is a good choice for them. If this is so, they should consider telling their doctors before surgery that if the ovaries are normal they should not be removed. This is discussed at greater length in the next chapter.

Some women who do not have distressing symptoms with fibroids are advised by their doctors to have the uterus removed (hysterectomy), simply because 'it is no longer a useful organ after childbearing is over'. In such situations it is a good idea to seek a second opinion from another doctor, and to remember that the uterus will shrink significantly in size after the menopause. Often it is possible to avoid a hysterectomy by waiting, thereby avoiding the risk and pain of this operation.

Some fibroids, however, enlarge to the size of a five-month pregnancy or more, which can cause significant abdominal swelling and may place uncomfortable pressure on the bladder or bowel. Fibroids can also cause very heavy menstrual bleeding, which may result in severe anaemia or make it difficult for a woman to carry on her daily activities. Profuse bleeding is often the result of so-called submucous fibroids, which lie just below the uterine lining and distort the normal shape of the uterine cavity. Any woman with very heavy periods should take supplemental iron, and ask her doctor to check her blood count at regular intervals. Sometimes medicines will help to check heavy bleeding. However, if the bleeding or other symptoms from fibroids are severe, the woman may opt for some kind of surgery. A variety of surgical treatments are currently available.

If the woman wants to retain her uterus and her fertility, she can choose a myomectomy, a surgical operation in which the fibroids are removed but the uterus remains. This operation requires considerable technical skill on the part of the gynaecologist, since it is important that all fibroids be removed, including very small ones that may be hard to detect. On rare occasions the operation becomes so technically difficult that the gynaecologist is forced to do a hysterectomy after all, removing the entire uterus. After a myomectomy (or a hysterectomy) there is a four-to-six-week recovery period before the woman has regained all her former strength. And there is a chance that the fibroids may grow back in future years, although this risk diminishes as the woman approaches her menopause. If menstrual bleeding was very heavy before a myomectomy, this situation is often improved after the operation. If the woman becomes pregnant, she may need to have a caesarean section for the delivery of the baby if the uterus has been significantly weakened by the myomectomy surgery. Myomectomy operations have become much more popular in recent years, as more women are waiting until 35 or 40 to have children, or are opting to retain their reproductive organs even if they don't want children.

Women with very heavy menstrual bleeding who want the most minimum surgery have another option, a new technique which uses a surgical laser. The laser beam destroys the uterine lining, removing most of it on a permanent basis so that little or no menstrual bleeding returns. The woman can no longer have children after this procedure. However, the rest of the uterus remains intact, and the recovery period after this surgery is much quicker – the patient leaves the hospital within one day. A similiar result is obtained with the use of an instrument called a resectoscope, which cuts away the uterine lining but leaves the rest of the uterus intact. Not all gynaecologists have been trained in using these new techniques – women who are interested should ask their doctor about this.

Some women with fibroids are happy to have their uterus removed. Heavy and painful menstrual periods, fatigue and weakness from the resultant anaemia, or pelvic pain from other complications such as past uterine infections or endometriosis can make hysterectomy a welcome option. Women who are seriously considering hysterectomy should take several steps in advance whenever possible. One is to discuss with their doctor the question of retaining their ovaries if the ovaries seem normal at the time of surgery. This allows for the continued production of ovarian hormones – oestrogen, progesterone, and androgens in the premenopausal years – and thus a smoother transition into menopause when that time comes. Even after menopause the ovaries continue to secrete androgenic hormones; the importance of these hormones throughout life is discussed in the next chapter.

Another question to discuss with your doctor is banking your own blood in advance, so that it can be used if you need a transfusion. If you are not anaemic you can bank several units of blood in the month before your operation, thereby insuring that you will not contract any virally transmitted diseases that are occasionally hard to detect in donated blood, such as hepatitis or AIDS. The blood supply in the United Kingdom is currently well screened, so that the risk of contracting such diseases through a transfusion is very low. However, many people are deciding to bank their own blood in advance of elective surgery, to be absolutely safe.

The decision of whether or not to have a hysterectomy is a complex one, especially if the operation is not really medically necessary. To clarify this point, a hysterectomy is often medically necessary for cancer, serious bleeding, overwhelming infection, severe pain, or other difficult problems. It is less necessary, or even optional, in many cases of fibroids or irregular bleeding that respond well to progestogens. Women facing a hysterectomy should discuss this fully with their doctors, making sure all their questions are answered. They should also be aware that there are emotional implications in surgery of any kind, some negative and some positive. Many fear the idea of losing a part of their body, entering a hospital with its relative impersonality, and experiencing pain, weakness, and possible complications from surgery. Others see drama in the hospital atmosphere and enjoy the special attention and the mind-altering drugs they receive. Some people who dread an operation in advance feel greatly helped by it in the long run, while others feel angry or assaulted by their surgical experience. Much of this depends on the skill and caring of the doctors and nurses who attend them, and the outcome of the surgery on their health. As there are many unpredictables in this situation, it is best to have it well thought through in advance.

CANCER OR OVERGROWTH OF THE UTERINE LINING

Unusually heavy, irregular, or persistent bleeding before the menopause, or bleeding that occurs unexpectedly after periods have stopped for six months or more, may be due to cancer or overgrowth of the lining of the uterus. If blood loss is excessive or if cancer is suspected, doctors recommend a D and C, usually to identify problems like polyps (usually benign, pod-shaped growths) or hyperplasia. Hyperplasia is not cancer, but a condition of over-activity of the lining cells. Occasionally cancer of the uterine lining is found, and surgical removal of the uterus (hysterectomy) is recommended, along with other treatments.

However, much of the time the diagnosis is some stage of hyperplasia, which can usually be treated with a progestogen, a medicine similar to progesterone. Progestogens inhibit overgrowth of the uterine lining and restore a normal pattern to the cells when taken for 10 to 14 days each month. If your doctor has suggested a hysterectomy for a non-cancerous condition such as hyperplasia, you can ask for a few courses of progestogens, followed by another D and C to assess the results. Sometimes the condition clears up very easily this way.

CANCER OF THE CERVIX

Sometimes irregular bleeding is caused by cancer of the cervix (the lower part of the uterus at the top of the vagina). The problem is easily diagnosed by a cervical smear taken during a pelvic examination, which should be continued regularly during the menopausal years. Cervical cancer is preceded for several years by a condition known as dysplasia of the cervix, also identified by cervical smears. Dysplasia of the cervix is not cancer, but a pre-cancerous condition of increased cellular activity, which sometimes becomes cancerous and sometimes returns to the original normal conditions. Dysplasia almost never occurs in women who have never had intercourse, and is rare in women who always use a condom or diaphragm during sex, since the abnormality of dysplasia and cervical cancer is initiated by some factor that comes from a male sexual partner. This factor is suspected to be a sexually transmitted virus, probably the wart virus.

Women with dysplasia or cancer of the cervix should obtain prompt medical treatment, which may include further diagnostic tests, freezing or laser treatment of the cervix, removal of part of the cervix, or hysterectomy. If a hysterectomy is not required, shielding the cervix with a condom or diaphragm in every act of intercourse will minimize further exposure to the initiating factor. If the woman is a smoker, giving up smoking will also reduce the risk, since several studies have shown a relationship between cigarette smoking and cervical cancer.

We have seen that bleeding problems in the menopause are variable and affected by many factors. Some women have virtually no bleeding problems and others have erratic episodes of spotting or flooding or both. Since some bleeding difficulties are caused by serious problems such as uterine cancer, it is wise to consult with your doctor regularly. On the other hand, it is encouraging to remember that the vast majority of bleeding problems in the menopause are the result of irregular ovulation and will be self-limiting. The best method of prevention is paying attention to healthy living from day to day, as discussed in the second half of this book (Chapter 12 onwards).

POSITIVE ASPECTS OF THE MENOPAUSE

The menopause is not always a problem – let's remember the positive aspects of this transition. After the menopause there are no more menstrual cramps, bleeding problems, or tampons and pads. There are no more aching pelvic discomforts with and after ovulation, no more tender breasts before a period, and no more mood swings with premenstrual tension. There are no more problems with fibroid tumours, birth control, or unwanted pregnancy. Migraine headaches tend to disappear. Not all women experience all these aggravations, but most have had some of them. Freedom from these difficulties is an aspect of the menopause to be enjoyed.

3.
THE OVARIES
– HIDDEN
SOURCES OF
WELL-BEING

Janet, a 45-year-old nurse, wanted a hysterectomy because of very large fibroid tumours that were causing pressure on her bladder. Her doctor said he would also remove both ovaries as a precautionary measure against ovarian cancer later on. 'You're almost in the menopause,' he said, 'so your ovaries won't be useful that much longer anyway.' 'Wait a minute,' answered Janet, 'I've always liked what my ovaries have done for me. If they look normal, I want you to leave them in.' Janet felt good about her decision, as she had read quite a lot about the low risk of cancer of the ovaries and the importance of these organs for general health and well-being. Her doctor found her ovaries were normal and did not remove them. Janet had a smooth recovery from her hysterectomy without needing to take any replacement hormones.

Throughout our lives our ovaries produce various hormones – oestrogen, progesterone, and androgens – which influence general health, bone structure, sexuality, and reproduction. The ovaries also produce a tiny egg cell each month during the menstrual years which can develop into a baby when fertilized by a sperm.

As a woman approaches the menopause these egg cells are

produced less regularly. This causes changes in the timing and amount of her menstrual flow, as we discussed in the previous chapter. Finally, around the age of 50, no further egg cells are released. The woman's ability to bear children has ended.

At the menopause, when the ovaries are no longer producing egg cells, the secretion of oestrogen and progesterone decreases greatly. However, the ovaries still play an important role at this time, because they continue to produce androgens, which influence general health and sexuality. Recent research indicates that androgens are secreted in small amounts even by women in their eighties. These hormones are similar to male hormones, but definitely belong in a woman's body. They help in maintaining muscular strength and sex drive. They help to keep the vagina elastic and lubricated. Androgens are also secreted by the adrenal glands, located above the kidneys. This adrenal output of androgens ensures that even women without ovaries produce some of these beneficial hormones.

Some androgens are converted to oestrogen in the body's fat cells, so women with more fat on their bodies produce more oestrogen after the menopause, and may have fewer problems with hot flushes, vaginal dryness, and brittle bones. Here at last is an advantage in being fat!

But, as usual, the middle way is best. Being too fat has discomforts and hazards, including the risk of producing too much oestrogen, which can cause cancer of the uterus (see Chapter 10). The best post-menopausal body is probably one that is a little plump, but still active.

In the past many doctors felt they should routinely remove the ovaries of a woman over 40 if they had to remove her uterus. They reasoned that in the menopause and beyond, the ovaries were useless organs which might become cancerous. The chance of a woman contracting cancer of the ovary in her lifetime is about 1% (it's lower in women who have borne children or taken the oral contraceptive pill, higher where there's a strong family history of ovarian cancer). Cancer of the ovary is hard to detect early and difficult to cure. Doctors reasoned that since they could give women

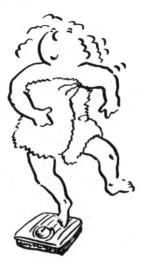

oestrogen pills to replace the hormones secreted by the ovaries, women would be better off without these organs.

New findings about post-menopausal ovaries are causing many doctors to change their views on the routine removal of healthy ovaries along with the uterus. The various hormones secreted by the ovaries in middle and old age contribute to well-being in many ways, and cannot always be duplicated by pills. For example, after ovarian removal some women find oestrogen pills do not restore their sex drive or their strength and well-being. They must also take androgen pills to fully regain their sexual interest, and thereby run the risk of growing excess hair and experiencing other side effects.

The argument for retaining the ovaries whenever possible should be balanced by the statement that in some cases the ovaries must be removed in surgery. For example, if they do contain cancer, very large benign cysts, infection, or if they are a source of chronic pain, their removal may enhance a woman's health and chances for survival. Any patient facing a hysterectomy should discuss this question carefully with her doctor.

However, this discussion may not be easy. Many gynaecologists still believe in the routine removal of ovaries after the age of 45 or 50, and some frighten their patients by saying they may get ovarian cancer if the ovaries are retained. Women faced with this dilemma should look carefully at their own situation, and ask a lot of questions. Unless there is a family history of frequent ovarian cancer, the chances of getting this disease are less than 1%. If the ovaries are not diseased they will continue secreting androgens for the rest of a woman's life, which will help her bones, muscles, sex drive, and general well-being. If her gynaecologist will not listen carefully to a woman's concerns in this matter, she may need to seek a second or third opinion. While it is difficult to be at odds with your doctor, your wishes for your own body need to be respected.

THE MENOPAUSE WITH OVARIES BUT NO UTERUS

A woman who has had her uterus removed in her thirties or forties, but still has her ovaries, may wonder how she will know when her 'change of life' is occurring. When should she expect hot flushes? What if she never gets hot flushes? How will she know when to apply the principles discussed in this book, such as taking extra calcium, exercising, or considering hormone replacement?

Generally a woman with ovaries but no uterus goes through the menopausal transition like other women. She has no more periods but her ovaries continue to function like other women's until her late forties. At that time, when she ceases to ovulate regularly and produces less oestrogen, she becomes aware of hot flushes, night sweats, and decreased vaginal secretions. If she has few symptoms of this kind (about 20% of women never get hot flushes) she can be fairly sure she has passed through the menopausal change somewhere between the ages of 48 and 53.

Hormone therapy can be considered when symptoms occur at the age of 50, whichever comes first. But no one should wait until a specific age to start exercising or eating foods high in calcium (see Chapter 7). Exercise is a good idea every day at every age. Calcium-rich foods are important for women throughout life, and calcium supplements can be started at 35 and then doubled at the age of 50 (see Chapter 16).

4.
HOT FLUSHES AND HOW TO SURVIVE THEM

Hot flushes are something like adolescent acne – an outward sign of a natural process of hormonal change that all women go through as they age. We need to accept ourselves and each other in this phase of life, with open discussions and a sense of humour.

Women become more sensitive to temperature around the time of the menopause. They often feel both cold and heat more acutely, and find they are frequently adding or removing sweaters. As menstrual periods cease, about 80% of women begin to experience hot flushes – feelings of extreme heat that come on unexpectedly. During a hot flush, the face, upper body, or entire body becomes very warm and flushed. Usually this feeling lasts for two or three minutes, but it can last longer – flushes continuing for an hour have been reported by some women. Sweating will also occur – sometimes a little and sometimes a lot. Before a flush begins, a woman often feels it coming. She may need to take off her coat or sweater and fan herself, which is understandable since her skin temperature suddenly rises 3° to 4° Centigrade (7° to 8° Fahrenheit). However, the temperature inside the body does not rise, and no fever occurs. Shortly after a hot flush the body temperature actually falls a little.

When hot flushes come at night, a woman may wake with feelings of breathlessness and heat. She often throws off the covers for a short time, and may sweat a small or large amount. Waking with frequent flushes may interrupt her sleep, which may in turn produce fatigue and difficulty concentrating during the day. Fortunately, these severe symptoms do not last long with most women, and sounder sleep is usually restored after 6 to 12 months.

In general, hot flushes are most intense and frequent in the first two years of the menopause, and then decrease in number and strength as the body gradually adapts to lower hormone levels and finds a new equilibrium. However, one-third of women still experience some feelings of heat as long as nine years after the menopause.

Hot flushes need to be demystified. While they can be uncomfortable if a woman is overdressed and cannot shed some clothing, they need not be accompanied by feelings of embarrassment, anxiety, or helplessness. The popular image of the middle-aged woman as an emotional wreck, drenched in sweat and unable to cope, has been played up by the pharmaceutical companies to persuade doctors and their patients to use drugs for this condition. For the younger woman this inaccurate image creates fear and dread of hot flushes. For the menopausal woman the most distressing aspect of a hot flush often is its visibility during the episode – her fear that others notice it and are making fun of or condemning her for growing older.

A discussion group was talking about hot flushes. Marie said that her appearance was very important in her job as a designer, and her hot flushes had made her very self-conscious. She was greatly relieved when her doctor prescribed oestrogen pills and the hot flushes went away. Sarah said that she had decided to live with the hot flush situation and had brought a small fan to work, so she could turn it on whenever necessary. Several younger women in her office had asked about it and appreciated her explanation of hot flushes. Susan said that she had had three intense hot flushes during the group discussion and she wondered how bad she had looked. There was a brief silence – no one had even noticed.

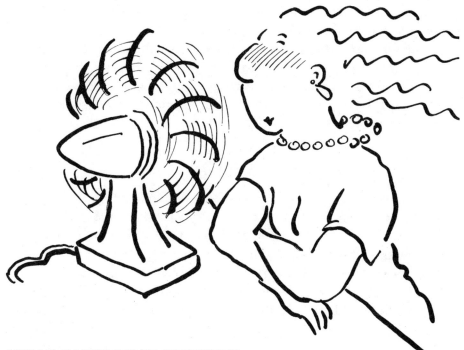

WHAT CAUSES HOT FLUSHES?

Hot flushes begin at a time in life when there is a relatively sudden decrease in oestrogen output from the ovaries. The more gradual the decrease, the less severe the symptoms. Some women with liberal amounts of body fat have fewer problems with hot flushes, because their fat tissues manufacture more oestrogen. On the other hand, very thin women or women who have had their ovaries removed surgically may have more difficulty with hot flushes. Smokers may also have more difficulty with hot flushes, because smoking reduces hormone output from the ovaries.

Although it is difficult to control or prevent hot flushes, women usually come to recognize precipitating factors. Hot drinks (especially coffee and tea), hot meals, alcohol, emotional upset, hot weather, a warm room, or a warm bed all can be triggers. Studies on the timing of hot flushes show them to be much more common between six and nine at night. Few flushes occur in the mornings on cool days, but many more occur in hot weather. All the precipitating factors mentioned here are directly or indirectly related to body temperature. Caffeine and food both raise metabolism and thereby warm the body. Alcohol causes skin flushing and makes us feel warmer. Emotional upset may do the same. Body temperature rises as the day goes on and is often at a peak in the early evening. A warm environment can also raise body temperature slightly.

WHAT'S BEHIND HOT FLUSHES?

The human body has several mechanisms to keep its internal temperature stable at an average 37° Centigrade (98.6° Fahrenheit). When the outside temperature is cold, we shiver and become pale. Shivering creates heat by contracting our muscles, and a pale skin signifies that the body is keeping our blood warmer by diverting its flow to deeper tissues, thus preventing its exposure to the cold world outside. When the outside temperature is warm, we sweat and flush, cooling ourselves as sweat evaporates and blood in the skin surface loses heat to the outside. Most people barely notice these mechanisms unless the temperature is extremely cold or hot. Menopausal women, however, flush and sweat in response to heat in an exaggerated way. Their core body temperature actually falls slightly after a flush, as might be expected, thus creating a need to put on a sweater shortly after taking it off!

Why do hot flushes occur in the menopause and beyond? Has the woman's internal thermostat changed in some way? Is this response related to a hormonal imbalance or state of deficiency, as many have alleged? Might it have some benefits, such as enabling older women to withstand the cold better? We do not know.

What we do know is that there is an area in the brain that regulates body temperature, keeping it in the range of 36° to 37°

Centigrade (97° to 99° Fahrenheit) despite wide shifts in outside temperatures. This 'thermostat' in the brain is adjacent to the area that governs the output of hormones by the pituitary gland and the ovaries. During the menopausal years the hormonal centre may influence and throw the 'thermostat' off balance, setting it lower and thus causing flushes and sweats to cool the body.

However, the story is more complex than this. Women who enter the menopause in their teens or early twenties, because of genetic reasons or surgical removal of the ovaries, rarely have hot flushes. Hot flushes occur in these women only if they take supplementary oestrogen for a time and then stop taking it. The trigger for hot flushes seem to be rapid withdrawal of oestrogen from a body that has grown accustomed to it. After a number of years this withdrawal effect is lessened and hot flushes become less frequent and intense.

LIVING WITH HOT FLUSHES

What does this tell us about living more easily with hot flushes? Since flushes accompany a rapid decrease in oestrogen, avoiding lifestyle factors that contribute to this problem will help. Smoking and excess alcohol interfere with ovarian function. Heavy use of marijuana and some other drugs may also affect hormonal output from the ovaries. Conversely, leading a healthy and drug-free life will permit the body to adjust more gradually to the menopausal process.

In addition, menopausal women should not be underweight. As explained in Chapter 3, oestrogen is actually manufactured in body fat from other hormones after the menopause. A very thin woman will have less natural oestrogen in her system, which may give her more problems with hot flushes.

Keeping cool is important for menopausal women, since all the precipitating factors in hot flushes are related to heat. Large meals, caffeine, alcohol, and strong emotions all make us warm. A menopausal woman reacts to heat by flushing and sweating in an exaggerated manner, so the most rational therapy for hot flushes is keeping cool. Don't overdress, keep the house cool, eat frequent small meals, and go easy on caffeine and alcohol. Take a cool drink of water or juice after exercise. All these things feel good and really help!

TREATMENT FOR HOT FLUSHES

If a woman is severely troubled by hot flushes, she has several choices. She can wait for the flushes to decrease over time, which will happen naturally, or she can consider taking oestrogen pills (hormone replacement therapy). The good news about oestrogen supplements is that they will quickly decrease or eradicate hot flushes in most women. The bad news is that hot flushes return whenever the drug is stopped. However, this return may be minimized if a woman tapers off her dose of oestrogen very slowly, over a period of months. The decision of whether or not to take oestrogen, with its various benefits and risks, is thoroughly discussed in Chapter 10 of this book.

Some doctors prescribe medicines other than oestrogen for hot flushes. A progestogen such as Provera, can be taken. These also decrease hot flushes, but not quite as effectively as oestrogen, and side effects like tiredness, weight gain, and depression can occur. Clonidine is available as pills and in skin patches which will last for up to a week. Low doses, 0.05 to 0.15 milligrams daily, are helpful to some women with severe hot flushes who should not or do not wish to take oestrogen thereapy. Clonidine is a prescription drug and should be used under the guidance of a physician familiar with its side effects. Other drugs that have been suggested for hot flushes include Catapres, a powerful medicine for lowering blood pressure which also causes a dry mouth, sedation and fatigue. In my opinion Catapres and tranquillizers should be avoided as a treatment for hot flushes – their use for this symptom has too many risks.

It is important to remember that all medicines that are effective have many effects on the body besides the one intended. This is also true of recreational drugs, many food and herbal remedies. Therefore, it is important to use any medicine wisely – only when needed, in the lowest effective dose, and for the shortest time that is necessary. Ask your doctor or chemist the reasons why any medicine is prescribed for you, and what its potential side effects are.

Some women are interested in alternative therapies, and try various combinations of herbal medicines or vitamins for menopausal symptoms. Popular books on the menopause have suggested that vitamin E in high doses, ginseng root, and other remedies are helpful. While there are many accounts of women who have been helped by these approaches, we do not yet have enough information on the doses and side effects involved. Like medicines, some may be helpful and others harmful. Prolonged use of high doses of ginseng, for example, has produced hypertension and other problems. All such therapies should be approached with common sense and a positive but careful attitude. Listen to the wisdom of your body, and discontinue any therapy that causes unpleasant, unbalanced feelings.

5.
SEX IN THE
SECOND HALF
OF LIFE

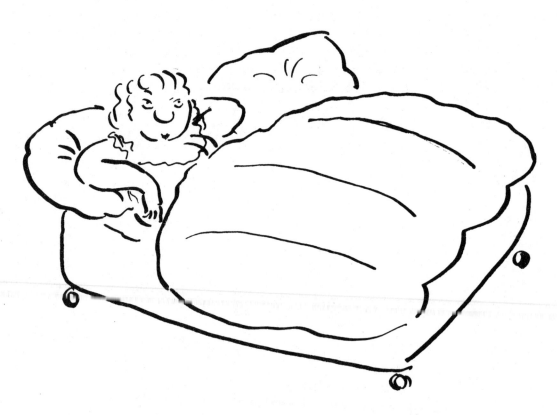

The nutty thing about being an older woman as far as sex is concerned is that most women don't feel old when it comes to sex.

Will the menopause mean the end of your sexuality? Not at all. The menopause is the end of a woman's fertility, or ability to become pregnant. However, she is still a sexual being capable of giving and receiving love in every way.

Sexual responsiveness changes with ageing in both women and men. The sex drive may seem less urgent and arousal may take longer. However, many women continue to be sexually active into old age, both with partners and by masturbating. What is true in youth is equally true for older people. There is a tremendous individual variation in sexuality. Some women report being less interested in sex after the age of 50, feeling other aspects of their lives are more important. Others say sex is more enjoyable than ever. Some women lack a sexual partner at this time in their lives, when men their age may have sexual problems or are more difficult to find. Some turn to other women for love and companionship. Many older women masturbate for sexual pleasure.

Many women have some degree of guilt about masturbation, even in midlife. They were probably taught in childhood that it was dirty or sinful to touch their genitals, and the resultant feelings of discomfort lingered on. Perhaps this guilt can be lessened by the realization that most people masturbate, and the practice is helpful in maintaining sexual responsiveness in midlife. Masturbation has helped many people at times when they had no suitable sexual partners. It may even have saved a few people from unsuitable partners!

VAGINAL DRYNESS AND LOVEMAKING

'I finally met a marvellous man,' said Diana. 'We were both taking evening classes at the local college. But when we got together to make love I felt extremely sore and I had to ask him to stop. He was worried he had hurt me and I've got to do something to improve this situation. I really like him!' I examined Diana, who was 52, and found that her vaginal mucous membranes were thin and tender. I explained to her that she needed to use a small amount of oestrogen cream on a regular basis, and a lubricant for intercourse. A few weeks later I bumped into Diana and she looked radiant. 'That situation is so much better,' she said. 'I feel really great again.'

The most frequent problem women in their fifties notice during intercourse is vaginal dryness and soreness. As oestrogen levels drop during the menopause and beyond, the vaginal walls become thinner and drier. The cervix no longer secretes the quantities of mucus it did during the fertile years. The entrance to the vagina becomes smaller, especially in a woman who has not borne children. As a result, intercourse can feel painful, even though a woman is sexually responsive and can easily achieve orgasm through stimulation of the clitoral area with the hand or mouth. Lesbian women usually have less difficulty with this problem because they may not use vaginal penetration in lovemaking, or may use a small object like a finger.

Several approaches are helpful. Couples should use lubricants during foreplay and wait until the woman is thoroughly aroused before vaginal penetration. Useful lubricants are creams (unscented or scented), vegetable oils, or water-soluble jellies such as K-Y. If the couple uses the woman-on-top position, she can control the rate of insertion of the man's penis and minimize any discomfort. Many women report that regular sexual activity, either masturbation or intercourse, helps reduce vaginal soreness. If these methods are not successful, a woman should talk to her doctor about using oestrogen creams (sese Chapter 10). These preparations are very helpful in promoting thickening of the vaginal lining, thereby reducing frictional discomfort or pain. Used in small doses under medical supervision, they can be very effective in eliminating the problem. If oestrogen cannot be prescribed for some reason, a cream containing 1% or 2% testosterone is often helpful.

A recent study of women after the menopause revealed that those who continued to have intercourse, or to masturbate, showed fewer signs of vaginal ageing than sexually inactive women. The women who continued intercourse had similar oestrogen levels but higher androgen levels than those who did not. The study appears to underline two important points. Firstly, that continuing to be sexually active through intercourse or masturbation may help to preserve vaginal function after the menopause. Secondly, that the ovaries – a major source of androgen secretion – remain active organs into old age.

What can couples do when their usual sexual activities become a problem? Frequently with ageing the man may have more difficulty getting and keeping an erection, or the woman with vaginal soreness. Illness or tiredness may impair the sexual response of one or both partners. Alcohol, tranquillizers and many medications can reduce sex drive and alter men's abilities to keep an erection. These problems should be discussed with a doctor, as some people can decrease or eliminate medicines by making changes in eating and drinking habits, increasing exercise, and learning how to relax.

It is also important for couples to realize that intercourse is not the only means of sexual expression. People give affection and pleasure to each other in many other ways, and can stimulate one another with their hands, mouths, or a vibrator, and through massage with oils and creams. While the urgency to achieve orgasm may decline with age, the gratification of giving and receiving a loving touch remains strong. Learning how to give and receive a slow, deep massage of the hand, foot, shoulders, or entire body is a wonderful experience at any age.

One of the problems with sex in younger years for many women is the lack of prolonged caressing and foreplay, and the rapidity with which sexual encounters lead to intercourse. In later life there is an opportunity to correct this imbalance. Instead of giving up on sex, couples can include more touching in their lives, more hugs, massage, and baths together. They can expand their definition of sensual pleasure.

KEGEL'S EXERCISES

Contracting and relaxing the muscles that surround the anus, vagina, and urethra (the opening for urine) can be very helpful. Women have found that these simple exercises increase their

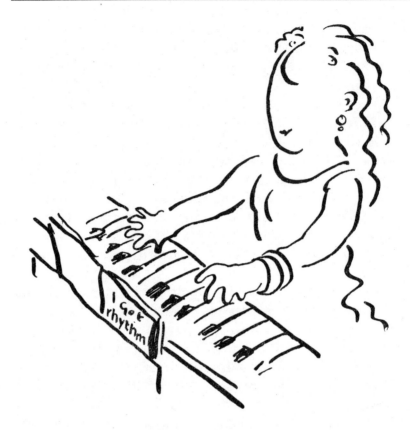

awareness of how to relax or to use these muscles during sex. Many have reported that it is easier to achieve orgasm after practising Kegel's exercises. Other women say they have less tendency to develop haemorrhoids (piles) or to leak urine while coughing, laughing, or sneezing.

Kegel's exercises, named after the gynaecologist who developed them to prevent urinary incontinence, are performed by imagining that you want to stop urinating, and squeezing the muscles in your vaginal area firmly. Practise this squeeze technique while counting to three, then relax. After repeating this squeeze-and-hold technique a number of times, try a rapid alternation between tightening and letting go of the muscles. You can perform these silent, simple exercises anywhere and anytime, while standing, sitting, or lying down.

IRRITATION, INCONTINENCE, AND INFECTION

Like the tissues lining the vagina, the lining of the urethra becomes thinner and less elastic after the menopause. Women may experience a need to urinate more frequently. Some have difficulty with leakage of urine when they cough, sneeze, or laugh. Urinary incontinence should be discussed with a doctor if it is severe. This can be treated with Kegel's exercises or in some cases with surgery.

As the vaginal tissues become thinner and drier after the menopause, they can easily be irritated by strong soaps. Warm (not hot) water is the best cleanser. For itching or irritated tissues, oatmeal baths are soothing (put some cooked oatmeal in a sieve and hold it under the tap as you fill the bath). Vaginal infections may occur after intercourse, especially with new partners, and often require a consultation with a doctor.

BIRTH CONTROL

How long should birth control methods be used in the menopausal years? As long as menstrual periods occur and, to be on the safe side, for the next 6 to 12 months. However, the likelihood of becoming pregnant around the age of 50 is small, so couples can use simple methods such as the diaphragm, sheath, or foam. An IUD, if already in place and comfortable, may be left in until periods stop, but should be removed if heavy bleeding or pain occurs. The pill should not be taken over the age of 40 in most cases, and not over 35 by smokers, because of the increased risk of complications such as a heart attack or stroke. Women following fertility awareness methods of birth control may have difficulty recognizing ovulation, which occurs less regularly and with less secretion of cervical mucus.

HYSTERECTOMY AND SEXUALITY

Women who are contemplating a hysterectomy for other than urgent reasons should get opinions from several doctors if possible, and should know that there are some sexual side effects from a hysterectomy.

While sexual pleasure leading to female orgasm is usually achieved from stimulation of the clitoris, the cervix and uterus also play a sexual role. To understand the sexual role of the uterus, we must think again about early theories on the female sexual response. Under the influence of Freudian theory, it was once believed that women who needed direct clitoral stimulation (as in masturbation or foreplay) to achieve orgasm were sexually immature. The 'completely sexual' woman responded to intercourse alone, according to this view, which emphasized the importance of the 'vaginal orgasm'.

Many sexologists in recent years have believed that all female orgasms originate in the clitoris, which may be stimulated directly by hand or mouth, or indirectly by intercourse. Vaginal penetration is not necessary for orgasm, and by itself may not provide enough indirect clitoral stimulation for high levels of arousal. Psychologists and feminists have used these findings to counter early Freudian theories, and debunk the 'myth of the vaginal orgasm'. Now our views are changing again on this controversial subject! For many women there is something about vaginal penetration (along with clitoral stimulation) that enhances the quality of sexual pleasure and orgasm. Instead of intercourse, some women use fingers or other objects to achieve these sensations.

The extra pleasure may come not only from the physical closeness of vaginal penetration, but from the stimulation of the cervix and uterus. After a hysterectomy, this is lost, as are the sensations from uterine contractions during orgasm. It is noteworthy that about one third of women who have had a hysterectomy report that their sexual pleasure decreased after surgery:

I had to have it all taken out, because I had a terrible infection from my IUD. But sex isn't quite the same as it used to be. I don't experience the same excitement at certain times of the month, and I miss the feeling of contractions deep inside. Still, I think I'm retraining myself to feel what I felt before by imagining what it used to feel like and trying to match it.

Women considering hysterectomy may be able to predict their own reactions in advance by self-observation. Women who find that cervical stimulation and/or deep thrusting greatly enhances the quality of their sexual pleasure may experience more loss after a hysterectomy. Conversely, those for whom deep penetration and movement in intercourse is painful may have better sex after a hysterectomy.

Until very recently, the uterus has been seen as primarily a reproductive organ without a sexual role. Now that we are more aware of its potential to enhance sexual experience, more research will appear to help women decide on the pros and cons of a hysterectomy. European gynaecologists have given more recognition to the sexual role played by the cervix and frequently perform a partial or subtotal hysterectomy when this operation is needed, removing the uterus but leaving the cervix and upper vagina intact. This operation has the added advantage of being simpler and quicker than a standard hysterectomy. However the woman must continue to have regular cervical smears to detect cervical cancer.

If both ovaries are removed at the time of a hysterectomy, a woman's sexual response is often changed. Oestrogen replacement by pill or injection will relieve hot flushes and prevent vaginal soreness, but it may not entirely restore the sex drive. It is not oestrogen, but androgenic hormones secreted by the ovaries and adrenal glands which make a woman feel more sexual. Androgens can be given by pill or injection, but they may cause increased facial hair growth, a lowered pitch of the voice, and liver damage if not carefully monitored. Small amounts of androgen cream have often been helpful (see Chapter 10).

These findings are causing many gynaecologists to reconsider the preventive removal of healthy ovaries during a hysterectomy, even in menopausal women. For many years it was believed that any decrease in sex drive women felt after such surgery was psychological, and that all problems could be solved by counselling and oestrogen. We are now less sure of these precepts and are coming to appreciate more the intricately connected wisdom of the body.

6.
YOUR LOOKS IN THE MENOPAUSAL YEARS

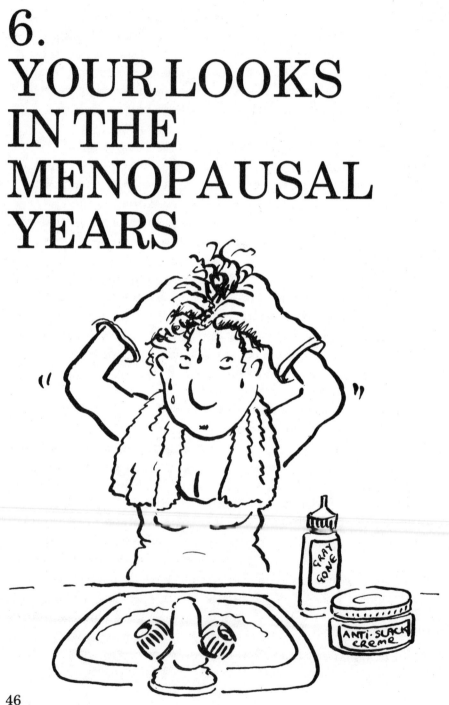

After her husband died Eileen felt neutered inside. She found she had lost interest in her appearance and in trying to relate to men. She had felt grey inside and out for several years until she met Jonathan in a folk dance class. He wasn't perfect and she would never marry him, but he helped her to feel alive again in an important way. She bought some new clothes and went to an exercise class. Her depression lifted and life began to glow. Her friends told her she looked wonderful. This is amazing, she said to herself. It's all still there, even at 55. This realization transformed her life in a subtle, positive way.

What will the menopause do to your looks? Will the hormonal changes leave you fat, wrinkled, stiff, and sexually unappealing?

Not necessarily. Women who have an early menopause due to surgical removal of the ovaries at 25, for example, still look 25 despite their hormonal loss. It is not the menopause but the ageing process that most affects our appearance. Ageing occurs at different rates in different people. Although genetic factors play a role in this, the crucial determinants of our appearance as we age seem to be health and happiness. We all get old and look old, but it can happen more or less beautifully, depending on our inner environment. Let's look at the questions about appearance.

WEIGHT GAIN

Weight gain can occur at the menopause but it is not necessarily inevitable. In our culture most people gain weight throughout their middle years because they exercise too little and eat too rich a diet. With ageing we tend to reduce body movement more than food intake. Before blaming this on the menopause, let's examine what role the sex hormones play in body weight.

Studies done on menstruating women show they are more active physically in the first two weeks after their periods, when oestrogen is the predominant hormone in their system. After ovulation, when progesterone is also produced by the ovaries, activity slows down and food intake increases. The body is preparing itself for pregnancy. Many women find they lose a little weight after

47

menstruation and then gain weight before their periods due to these hormonal influences. For women on the birth control pill, taking a progestogen with oestrogen for the whole month, weight gain is common.

But what about the menopause? At this time oestrogen levels fall sharply, and progesterone almost disappears from the system. Not only do we lose the subtle influence of oestrogen to stimulate physical activity, but also the progesterone effect which causes increased appetite and a slower pace. The net effect of the two hormones was to maintain weight levels, with a slight seesaw effect. After the menopause, the seesaw effect is gone, but there is no hormonal reason for continued weight gain. We are on our own, needing to balance food intake with exercise. This doesn't necessarily mean a stringent diet for the rest of our lives. It means eating lots of the right foods (whole grains, vegetables, fruit, and skimmed milk products) and as little as possible of the wrong foods (fats, sugars, refined flours, and rich meats). It means lots of walking, bending, and other movement. In societies where this happens naturally, many people become thinner after the menopause rather than fatter.

Women who take oestrogen after the menopause have been studied for the effect of this on their body weight. They have been found to weigh significantly less than women of a comparable age not on oestrogen. However, most of these studies so far have been done on older women taking oestrogen alone, without added progestogen. In recent years it has become apparent that a progestogen should be added to oestrogen in the last ten days of each month to minimize the cancer risk. Under these circumstances some weight gain may occur, which might minimize the differences between hormone users and non-users.

SKIN CHANGES

Another common concern about the menopause is that the skin will become rapidly dry and wrinkled. In younger women the sex hormones produced by the ovaries have various effects on the skin.

Oestrogen has the effect of liquefying the waxy material produced in skin cells and thereby reducing the severity of blackheads and acne. Androgens, also produced by the ovaries, make acne worse. After the menopause, when both hormones are reduced, facial pimples are rarely a severe problem but dryness and thinning of the skin due to the reduced amounts of fat beneath it often accompany ageing. The menopause does play a part in this process, but the changes are gradual.

The two most common causes of wrinkling and ageing of the skin are smoking and excessive exposure to sunlight. Smoking decreases the blood supply to the skin cells by constricting small blood vessels throughout the body. In addition, the blood of a smoker conveys less oxygen and more carbon monoxide than is normal. Skin cells and their underlying elastic layer are thus undernourished and lose their moisture and their natural contour, resulting in wrinkles. After the age of 30 or 35, the skin of smokers and non-smokers begins to look different. Next time you are on an aeroplane, notice the skin of people sitting in the non-smoking and smoking sections as you walk up and down the aisle. Wrinkles around the eyes, lines and creases, and a blue-grey colour due to poor oxygenation are all more apparent among smokers. The colour difference can be reversed when smoking is stopped, but the wrinkles remain.

Exposure to the sun is the most significant cause of skin wrinkling. People with brown or black skin are more protected from this effect and often have a smooth, youthful skin into old age. White people, with their lighter skin colouring, are more prone to skin damage from sun exposure. Sunburn damages the elastic layers underneath the skin cells, causing them to become less supportive. Fair-skinned people who work outdoors all their lives often have wrinkled, weather beaten skin. They also are more likely to develop skin cancer. Some sunshine is healthy and promotes vitamin D formation in the skin, but sunburn can cause problems. People with fair skin should wear hats and protective clothing or sunscreen lotions on bright days.

Finally, general health and nutrition affect our skin as we age.

Virtually all essential nutrients are needed for healthy skin. People who ignore the precepts of healthy eating and living but take large amounts of one or two vitamins or minerals are not helping their skin and appearance as much as people who eat a variety of whole natural foods and take a balanced vitamin/mineral supplement only when needed.

Many people know vitamin A plays a role in the health of skin and eyes. However, this fat-soluble vitamin can be stored in the body, and excessive amounts from animal sources or vitamin pills can be dangerous. Most people should not taken more than 15,000 IU (International Units) daily as a supplement. It is better to get most vitamin A from foods like carrots, sweet potatoes, yellow and red fruits, peppers, and all deep green, leafy vegetables.

Use of moisturizing skin cream is helpful for dry skin. Excessive hot water and soap wash away protective natural skin oils and should be avoided. Some cosmetics contain many chemicals which can be absorbed through the skin. Nothing will improve your appearance as much as a walk in the open air, healthy food, and activities that bring happiness and relaxation.

LOSS OF FLEXIBILITY

Changes in body flexibility – in the movement of the joints and the elasticity of the muscles – do occur with ageing, but can be counteracted with stretching and exercise. It is not the menopause that creates stiffness and joint pain so much as our habits of living, including insufficient movement, excess weight, and the wrong foods. A gentle programme of stretching exercises, such as yoga, and a daily walk can restore a flexibility.

SEX APPEAL

Many women worry about losing their sex appeal after the menopause. But sex appeal is a subtle force, made up of many variables, including interest in sexuality, transmitted verbally and by body language, and warmth and interest in others. These factors need not change with the menopause. There are, however, hormonal factors which act as subtle sex attractants in younger women. At the time of ovulation, when oestrogen levels are high, women secrete an odour which attracts men, even though they are not aware of the smell. These sex attractions are known as pheromones. Their effects can be easily seen in the animal world when a female is 'in heat' and fertile. Studies with human couples have shown that men initiate intercourse more often during a woman's fertile time. This source of sexual attraction is lost after the menopause. However, the use of subtle perfumes may stimulate the same areas in the brain as the pheromones did, giving out the same message of sexual receptivity. Among humans the most important sexual organ is the mind – most of our turn-ons and turn-offs are related to our thought processes. If you are interested in sexuality, you can be sure the menopause will not create a sudden end to your sex appeal.

The message of this chapter is that physical appearance does change with ageing, but not markedly with the menopause itself. The changes that come about with ageing are minimized by healthy living and a sense of meaning in life, which is why some old people look young and some young people look old.

7.
KEEPING YOUR BONES STRONG

Erica was worried about developing brittle bones, or osteoporosis. Her mother had lost considerable height with ageing and had back pain whenever she walked any distance. 'What can I do if I don't want to take oestrogen?' asked Erica. 'I've heard that lots of calcium and a vegetarian diet are helpful.' 'You're right about that,' I said 'Another thing you can do is to exercise every day.' 'I haven't really exercised in years,' groaned Erica. 'Isn't it dangerous to start suddenly?' 'Start with a short daily walk,' I suggested, 'and work up to 30 minutes a day at a brisk pace. Find something you really enjoy, like dancing or hiking, for the weekends. Start slowly and keep it up.'

After the menopause women are more likely to develop osteoporosis – a condition in which the bones lose their strength and fracture easily. 'Osteon' is the Greek word for bone, and 'porosis' means full of tiny holes or porous. Bones which have osteoporosis are more likely to break, bend, or become compressed, leading to pain and disability.

THE BIOLOGY OF OSTEOPOROSIS

Why do older women develop osteoporosis? Throughout life our bones are constantly being remodelled – they are not inert organs despite their apparent rigidity. At certain times calcium is dissolved out of our bones to replenish the calcium supply in the blood, and in this process bone becomes weaker. This happens when our diets are too low in calcium and when we are physically inactive. Reducing diets are often deficient in calcium and are responsible for bone loss in many women. At other times increased amounts of calcium enter the bones from the blood stream, making them denser, stronger, and larger. This happens when we do physical work and exercise, and also when there is plenty of calcium in our diets.

Calcium is a mineral with many functions. Besides giving strength to bones and teeth, it is dissolved in the blood and body fluids where it plays a role in muscle contraction, the functioning of the heart, the transmission of nerve impulses, and the blood-clotting system. The body has many glandular systems which regulate and stabilize the calcium level in the blood, pulling it in and out of the bones and in and out of our digestive tracts.

At the time of the menopause there is a steep drop in oestrogen production in women. Among its many functions, oestrogen plays a major role in helping the bones replenish their stock of calcium, thus preserving bone strength. When oestrogen is no longer abundant, the bones dissolve more rapidly than they recalcify, and a woman's bones may become softer, weaker, and therefore more likely to break. Why does oestrogen play such an important role in keeping our bones strong? No one is sure, but it is probably a mechanism to protect the bones from excessive calcium loss during pregnancy, and rapidly to replenish the calcium level in the bones between the end of breast feeding and the next pregnancy. At these times oestrogen levels in the body are high. While a woman is breast feeding her oestrogen levels are low and calcium leaves the bones to go into milk formation.

After the menopause, when oestrogen levels drop, about 25% of white, Asian, and brown-skinned women develop serious osteoporosis. Black women rarely develop this problem, for reasons we don't entirely understand. As a race blacks have thicker bones, which gives them a selective advantage against fractures. Susceptible women may fracture their wrists after a fall or even a knock – this commonly occurs in the fifties. In their sixties, women may experience back pain as a result of the loss of calcium in their spine, with 'crush fractures' or severe compression of vertebral bones. Loss of height and a humped back may result. While about 20% of women show vertebral compression by the age of 70, severe pain and disability is rare. Many women are not aware of having the condition. The most significant bone problem occurs typically after the age of 70 when fracture of the head of the thigh bone, commonly known as fracture of the hip, may take place. It is not uncommon for women living to the age of 80 to suffer from this condition and a small number of such patients will die from complications of the fracture. Those who recover are often permanently limited in their ability to walk without pain.

Osteoporosis can also cause tooth loss, which is more common in women than in men after the age of 50, and also more common in smokers. The weakened bone structure in the jaws of women with osteoporosis permits the loosening and ultimate loss of teeth.

Clearly there are significant problems associated with osteoporosis in some older women. How can we identify the 25% of women who are at risk of incurring fractures with ageing due to osteoporosis?

WHO'S AT RISK?

Medical scientists are working on screening tests to identify those at greater risk of fractures. At the time of writing, there is much debate but no agreement about the utility of *any* x-ray or laboratory tests to predict who is going to have osteoporotic fractures in the future.

A variety of x-ray techniques have been developed in recent years which are designed to screen women at the time of menopause, in order to identify those who are losing bone most rapidly and may therefore be most at risk of fractures. These tests may be helpful in predicting vertebral compression fractures of the spine, but are not considered useful in predicting hip fractures. One test commonly used is called dual-photon absorptiometry or DPA, which measures the density of bone in the vertebrae of the low back. The other test is the more widely known computed tomography or CT scan, which surveys the same vertebrae using a different radiological technique. While both tests have certain advantages and disadvantages, I prefer the DPA test as it subjects the patient to significantly less radiation than the CT scan. If a women has a bone screening test such as a DPA or CT at the onset of menopause and again a year later, the tests may help identify whether she is a rapid bone loser who could benefit from hormones, or a slow bone loser who might not need them to prevent subsequent vertebral crush fractures. However, it should be understood that these tests are subject to a certain percentage of errors, which makes it difficult for them to detect accurately small changes in bone density. At present they are not considered truly predictive for fractures – they only indicate an increased or decreased risk based on preliminary data. Many women with low bone density avoid fractures, and some with high bone density sustain them.

Because of the growing interest in osteoporosis, many new programmes designed for mass screening with DPA or CT have been developed and promoted in recent years. However, since the information collected so far does not allow accurate predictions of who will have a fracture, it is not ethical to advocate that large numbers of midlife women take these tests.

Biochemical tests for prediction of rapid bone loss after menopause are also under evaluation, and promise to be less expensive than x-ray studies. Measurements of body fat, oestrogen levels in the blood, and the excretion of calcium or other products in the urine, calculated in a special way, can all be helpful in determining who may be at risk. Women with more body fat tend to have higher oestrogen levels and less problem with brittle bones! At present most of these tests are only beginning to be used, so their validity in predicting fracture rates is still under investigation. We will be hearing more about these tests in coming years, which will help doctors and women decide who is most at risk.

Because of the lack of tests that can validly predict fracture risk, most thoughtful doctors rely on genetic and lifestyle factors – such as race, body build, and use of alcohol or cigarettes – to help decide who is most at risk from brittle bones. The table below summarizes these factors, which will be discussed individually. Read the table with care, noting how it applies to you individually.

FACTORS THAT INCREASE YOUR RISK OF OSTEOPOROSIS AND FRACTURES

Genetic or Medical Factors	Lifestyle Factors
Being in a non-black ethnic group	High alcohol use
Previous fractures that occurred easily, without major trauma	Smoking
Female relatives with osteoporosis	Lack of exercise
Being thin (especially if you are short)	Low-calcium diet
Early menopause (before age 40)	Lack of vitamin D from sun, diet, or pills
Chronic diarrhoea or surgical removal of part of the stomach or small intestine	Very high-protein diet
Kidney disease with dialysis	High-salt diet
Daily use of cortisone	Never having borne children
Daily use of thyroid extract (over two grains), Epanutin or aluminium containing antacid drugs	High caffeine use (e.g. over five cups of coffee or tea daily)

(Factors below line in each list are less important than those above it.)

Genetic And Medical Factors: All ethnic groups except blacks are at risk for osteoporosis. Black women rarely develop the problem, perhaps because of heavier bones or favourable hormonal differences.

Women who have had a previous fracture that occurred easily – from a minor fall, light blow, or twisting movement – may already have some osteoporosis.

Women with female relatives who had fractures or significant height loss with ageing may inherit a family tendency toward osteoporosis.

Women who are slim, with small muscle mass, are more at risk of osteoporosis than heavier, more muscular women. This is especially true if they are short and thin, as their total body weight is less. Several reasons are obvious here – more weight means more gravitational pull on the body and more work for the bones and muscles – all of which keep the calcium level in the bones high. More fat means more oestrogen production within the body which helps prevent osteoporosis (see Chapter 3). The slender smoker is at greatest risk, and the obese non-smoker at lowest risk of bone fractures.

Women with an early menopause often have more osteoporosis, since they lose bone over a longer period of time.

Patients with chronic diarrhoea, such as ulcerative colitis or Crohn's disease, absorb less calcium and lose more in their stools. The same problems can occur if part of the intestinal tract has been removed by surgery. Patients on kidney dialysis can develop calcium deficiency and need special care for this problem. Patients who use cortisone daily in significant amounts develop osteoporosis. Women on high daily doses of thyroid extract may develop osteoporosis, although the evidence for this is incomplete. Epanutin antacid drugs are other medicines that can cause loss of bone calcium.

Lifestyle Factors: Let's look at lifestyle – the daily habits that cause osteoporosis, as well as those that increase bone strength.

High alcohol use contributes to osteoporosis and bone fractures. Excess alcohol is toxic to the ovaries, causing infrequent ovulation and menstrual irregularities in younger women, as well as decreased breast size. The menopausal woman who uses alcohol heavily may have less hormonal output from her ovaries, and as a result will have more problems with hot flushes, vaginal soreness, and rapid loss of calcium from her bones. Many people who drink heavily do not pay attention to their diets, which compounds the problem of loss of calcium from the bones. Finally, heavy use of alcohol leads to accidents, falls, and fractures.

Smoking contributes to osteoporosis. First of all, smokers have a decreased oestrogen output and an early menopause. Several studies have shown significantly higher rates of bone fractures in post-menopausal smokers, probably because of the harmful effects of smoking on the ovaries and other glands, including the parathyroid glands in the neck which regulate calcium levels in the blood. Since smokers tend to weigh less and exercise less than non-smokers, their risk of osteoporosis is higher on this account. Thin smokers have a high risk of fractures.

Lack of exercise can cause osteoporosis. When people are inactive during illness, their bones will lose calcium just as their muscles will become weaker. Conversely, when we walk, run, jump, dance, or otherwise jar our skeletons, a mild electrical charge develops along the bone which stimulates bone growth and calcification. This electrical charge is sometimes used by orthopaedic surgeons to promote more rapid healing of fractures, by running a very low electrical current along the shaft of an injured bone. Our arms as well as our legs need exercise to keep our bones strong. Tennis players have significantly thicker bones in the arm that holds the racket. Thicker bones in the arms can be achieved through energetic swimming, gardening, lifting, callisthenics and pushups, weight training, and other similar exercise. Jogging or walking while moving the hands holding small weights is also useful.

A very interesting study was done at the University of Wisconsin by Dr Everett Smith. He studied women in a nursing home, average age 80, by measuring the size of their bones and the level of calcium in them with an x-ray technique. One group of women exercised their arms and legs for 30 minutes three times a week *sitting in their chairs*, a second group took extra calcium, and a control group made no changes in their diet and exercise. While the control group lost bone calcium during the three years of the study, the exercise group and the calcium group both gained bone, the exercise group most of all. When you consider that these women were about 80 years old and exercised from their chairs, the results are very encouraging. Think how much more we can achieve at a younger age with a more vigorous programme! Clearly, part of the current problem of osteoporosis is related to our sedentary lives and our reliance on motorized transport instead of our feet. Women who leave all the 'heavy work' to men are not using their bodies enough or doing the best for their bones. Exercise should be a lifelong commitment, planned for every day. Chapter 14 gives more suggestions on how to begin and maintain an enjoyable and self-perpetuating exercise routine.

A low-calcium diet can also contribute to osteoporosis. Elderly people who subsist on tea, toast, luncheon meat, and canned fruit may be in short supply of calcium. International studies have shown that countries with a low-calcium diet, like Japan, have more problems with osteoporosis and fractures than countries with a high-calcium diet, like Finland.

Calcium is contained in many common foods which should be consumed regularly by midlife women (as well as younger women who are pregnant or lactating). As the table on page 61 shows, a wide variety of foods are good calcium sources. You can still get plenty of calcium even if you don't like milk products.

Many other foods are also good sources of calcium. However, spinach, chard, parsley, rhubarb, and chocolate are not included here since the calcium in them is poorly absorbed.

In addition to paying attention to calcium in the diet, women should take calcium supplements after the menopause. It is widely recommended that women take 800 milligrams to one gram of elemental calcium daily. Some have suggested that this practice begin at the age of 35, so women will enter the menopause with bones of maximum strength. When calcium tablets are taken regularly for several years, there is evidence that older women can actually gain bone strength rather than continue to lose it. Calcium tablets, and foods containing calcium, are best taken in divided doses rather than all at once, to enhance absorption. Calcium in the form of calcium lactate, gluconate or carbonate is easily found in chemists and health food stores. Some samples of calcium from bonemeal and dolomite have contained lead and other contaminants and are not currently recommended.

Whether a high-calcium diet at the time of menopause will protect against bone loss is debatable. Ideally, the high calcium intake should have started many years earlier, to enable women to reach menopause with maximum bone strength. When oestrogen levels drop off at menopause, bone loss is accelerated in most women. Calcium supplements started at this time have not been shown to protect the bones of the vertebral spine, but do have some protective effect on the long bones of the legs and arms. This protective effect is maximized if oestrogen is also taken, as explained in Chapter 10.

Vitamin D must be present in the body to allow the absorption of calcium from the intestine. This vitamin is formed on the skin when it is exposed to the sun and it is stored in the liver until needed. However, many people are cut off from direct sunlight by clothing, remaining indoors, long dark winters, window glass, or smog. Others rightly fear that excess exposure to the sun may cause skin cancer or more rapid ageing of the skin. For these reasons vitamin D has been added to many milk products. Older women should get about 400 IU (International Units) of vitamin D daily to ensure optimum calcium absorption. This is most easily done by taking a daily multivitamin supplement containing vitamin D. Excess vitamin D (over 400 IU daily) is not advisable – this vitamin should be taken in 'megadoses' only in very few medical conditions.

A very high-protein diet is one which contains twice the body's daily needs for protein – ham and eggs for breakfast and meat, fish, poultry, or dairy products at other meals. Eating like this is common in Western countries. Many people consider such food indispensable for health, and a symbol of good living. Dieters often subsist mainly on protein-rich foods. While small amounts of protein are essential, large amounts can cause problems. Animal foods are often high in fat and can lead to obesity and heart disease. In addition, they play a role in the osteoporosis story. The end products of digesting protein-rich foods are acids such as sulphuric acid, which the body excretes in urine. In response, the kidneys

COMMON FOODS HIGH IN CALCIUM

Skimmed milk powder	Tahini (sesame seed paste)
Low-fat milk	Kale, cooked
Yogurt	Salmon, canned with bones
Low-fat cottage cheese	Broccoli, cooked
Cabbage greens, cooked	Tofu (soya bean curd)
Sardines, canned	Corn tortillas
Molasses	

Also, when making soup stock from bones, add one or two tablespoons of vinegar during the boiling process. The acid in the vinegar will dissolve the calcium out of the bones, providing a soup stock unusually rich in calcium.

excrete calcium to balance this acid. Even young people eating a very high-protein diet lose significant amounts of calcium in their urine. The post-menopausal woman is most at risk from this dietary cause of calcium loss, because of her lack of oestrogen with its protective effect on bones.

Bone studies on elderly women eating high-meat diets, mixed diets, and vegetarian diets, show that high-meat eaters have the most osteoporosis, and vegetarians the least. Nutritional research indicates that the post-menopausal woman should not emphasize flesh foods, but concentrate on eating whole grains, beans, vegetables, fruits, and skimmed or low-fat milk products. In middle age and beyond, women and men will be healthier if they try new answers to the question, 'What's for dinner?' Try some of these answers – baked potatoes and a big salad with bean sprouts and toasted sesame seeds, or split pea soup with wholewheat bread and cheese, or curried mixed vegetables with brown rice and yogurt. Sounds good?

A diet high in salt (sodium chloride) is detrimental in several ways. It has long been known that too much salt can lead to high blood pressure in susceptible people. Recently it has also been found that salt has the effect of causing the kidneys to excrete more calcium in the urine. In the long run such urinary loss of calcium can contribute to osteoporosis. Dramatic decreases in urinary calcium have been documented in patients with kidney stones when they reduce their salt intake.

Women who have never had children have more risk of osteoporosis, because the high hormone output in pregnancy contributes to bone strength. While this is true in Western countries, where pregnancies are limited in number and dietary calcium is adequate, it is often not true in developing countries where numerous pregnancies and a poor diet can lead to bone weakness.

The relationship between heavy caffeine use and osteoporosis has only recently been studied. Caffeine is found in coffee, tea, Coca Cola and similar drinks, and some medicines. In high doses caffeine can increase calcium loss from the body. This effect is small if a person drinks only one or two cups of coffee or tea daily, but can be significant if strong coffee or tea is consumed all day long. Since caffeine has other negative effects on health, contributing to chronic anxiety, disturbed sleep, and possibly to breast cysts, it is best to use it sparingly. Many heavy coffee drinkers are also smokers, as these habits tend to be linked. Suggestions for giving up smoking are discussed in Chapters 15 and 17.

OESTROGEN AND OSTEOPOROSIS

Osteoporosis can be prevented almost entirely by the use of oestrogen tablets (hormone replacement therapy – see Chapter 10), beginning at the menopause and continuing for many years. Oestrogen is very effective in halting the process of bone thinning and promoting bone strength. Numerous studies have shown a reduction in bone fractures among women taking oestrogen tablets, and many doctors regard this medication as an important answer to the problem of bone loss with ageing. Others, however, point out that every powerful medicine has some adverse side effects, and it is not safe or feasible to treat all women with hormones. Better ways are needed to identify those most at risk of fractures and, ideally, offer them a choice of hormones or a high-calcium diet combined with exercise. Further studies are needed to clarify the relative advantages of these two approaches.

Women who cannot take oestrogen may use a progestogen tablet regularly to help prevent osteoporosis. These compounds are not quite as effective as oestrogen but do help to prevent bone loss and hot flushes. However, as explained in Chapter 10, their long-term side effects on the heart, blood vessels and breasts need more study.

Some researchers suggest that women should take fluoride supplements to retard bone loss, along with varying amounts of calcium, vitamin D, and oestrogen. Fluoride will help with the problem, but the suggested large doses have unacceptable toxicity and should not be used.

This has been a complex chapter because of the many factors that influence bone strength. In summary, some people are more at risk than others from fractures due to osteoporosis. As the table on page 55 shows, the woman most at risk is Asian or white, thin, with a family history of fractures with ageing, and an early menopause. These genetic risks are greatly increased if she smokes, drinks heavily, does not exercise, and eats a high-protein, low-calcium diet. Conversely, women of any genetic background can greatly decrease their risk of fractures with ageing by not smoking, exercising daily, eating high-calcium foods, taking calcium supplements with vitamin D, and minimizing meat, alcohol, salt, and caffeine in their diets. Finally, oestrogen and progestogen tablets can be taken after the menopause to prevent osteoporosis. The decision to take these hormones needs careful thought by a woman and her doctor because of their potential side effects, as discussed in Chapter 10. As soon as the pills are discontinued, the risk of bone loss returns. In any case, we never outgrow our need for healthy eating and body movement. The final choice, however, will often be a very personal one, as the following two cases illustrate.

Janice, at 53, felt more secure after she started taking oestrogen tablets to increase her bone strength. At 52 she had tripped in the street and fractured her ankle. The year before she broke her wrist when she fell downstairs. Slim and small, Janice had followed a high-protein reducing diet for years. She had difficulty digesting milk products. She had a sedentary job in a bank and rarely exercised beyond doing housework. She was happy to take oestrogen pills, as they seemed the easiest solution and they also ended her hot flushes.

Ruth knew that she did not want to take hormones after the menopause. She always tried to find natural remedies for physical problems and was not a believer in pills. She was determined to see the menopause as a natural part of life, and not get upset by it. When her doctor told her she needed more exercise, she began walking to and from work in tennis shoes. He also suggested that she chew mint flavoured calcium tablets at bedtime. She did some reading on the menopause and felt secure in her decision to let nature take its course.

8.
HORMONES AND EMOTIONAL IMBALANCE

Popular mythology depicts the menopausal woman as going a little off her rocker. Are there special psychological risks for menopausal women? Are they more prone to depression, anxiety, irritability, and a general inability to cope?

If a woman in her late forties gets angry or cries, her emotion is often blamed on 'the change of life', just as in her thirties it was blamed on her periods or pregnancy. This kind of thinking can make women feel helpless and at the mercy of their hormones. It often prevents them from examining the factors in their relationships, families or jobs that may well cause anger or depression.

One of my therapy groups was talking about their emotional responses to the menopause. 'The menopause has been a really hard time for me,' said Sally. 'I feel much more vulnerable and get depressed easily. I cry when my daughter leaves home or if my boss is unreasonable.' 'Listen, Sally,' said Pam, 'You're facing the classic midlife crisis in my opinion. You'll be living alone when your daughter gets married and if your boss fires you you're sunk!'

'It's too bad it all happens at once,' answered Sally. 'I have a hard time coping with hot flushes, my boss, and my daughter's leaving.' 'Something similar happened to me,' said Alice. 'Then I moved into a house with some friends and it got better. I am not lonely anymore and I'm better off. Actually I feel happier than I have in years – and I'm going through the menopause too!'

It is important to attempt to clarify the issues. Do the end of ovulation and the drop in hormone levels at the menopause create a psychological imbalance in some women, triggering depression, anxiety, or delusion? Or is the drop in hormone levels relatively neutral, psychologically speaking? Perhaps emotional upset during the menopause is caused by important coincidental changes in a woman's life, and the way middle age is viewed in our culture, rather than by hormonal changes.

These two views of the psychology of the menopause have been debated for some time, and the issues are complex and interrelated. In this chapter we will look at both sides, and attempt to extract what is valuable from the two different viewpoints.

It is important to say at the outset that no peak of emotional illness is found in the menopausal years. Surveys of women in their mid-forties to mid-fifties show that hot flushes and night sweats are the only symptoms *directly* related to the menopause. Other symptoms, such as depression, anxiety, headaches, or dizzy spells, occur in some women before, during, and after the menopause, without a peak at any specific age. Moreover these symptoms tend to occur together. Some women experience many such problems, while others have very few.

But what about women who do feel more anxious and depressed in their menopausal years? While they may be in the minority, how do we account for their problems, and what solutions are available? Can you predict whether you are more or less likely to experience this special kind of midlife crisis?

CULTURAL FACTORS

Let's examine first the viewpoint of those who say it is *not* our hormones but our psychological reactions to ageing and to outer circumstances that cause emotional problems in the menopause.

In our society women have been judged by their physical appearance more than anything else. The emphasis we place on beauty, fashion, figure, and youth makes it difficult for some women to value themselves as they become middle aged. This is especially true for those who used their glamour and sexiness to attract men and enhance their sense of self-esteem. It can be devastating for such a woman if her husband or lover leaves her for a younger mate, which sometimes happens in midlife. Even without this problem she may become upset over vaginal dryness and pain with intercourse, feeling she is inadequate or invalidated as a sexual partner. She may feel that the end of her fertility means the end of her sexuality, and no longer view herself as a desirable person. She may consider hot flushes an embarrassing, visible sign of ageing.

All these feelings can add up to anxiety and depression, which cause her to seek medical help. In most cases she will ask for or be given oestrogen tablets, which are quite effective in relieving vaginal soreness with sex and reducing hot flushes. If this makes her feel better, we don't conclude that oestrogen is an antidepressant, but that oestrogen relieved her physical symptoms, thereby providing her with a good psychological lift.

Not all women react to ageing with depression, despite the cultural pressures that reward youthful female beauty and sexiness. Women who value themselves in their work, or as friends or family members, have an easier time adjusting to the waning of youth. They may see the menopause as a welcome end to menstrual periods, and accept its bodily changes as normal. They go through the same hormonal process as the woman who becomes distraught, but they interpret it differently.

When children leave home for jobs, college, or marriage, mothers may have problems with this loss which are blamed on the menopause. Actually, this change can occur when a woman is in her thirties or her sixties, depending on when the youngest child leaves home. And despite all the mythology about the 'empty nest', most parents feel quite positive about their children's maturity. Some women, however, do feel they have lost a major reason for existence – this is especially true of women who have focused their energies primarily on their children. Feelings of anxiety and depression about the loss of the mother role can be very painful. So can feelings of guilt about parenting, if children's lives are disturbed by illness, drugs, unwanted pregnancy, or failure in school or work.

If the woman's anxieties are blamed on the menopause, solutions are often sought in an oestrogen pill or a tranquillizer, and the real issue is left untouched. It is important for such women to re-examine what they want to do with their lives beyond mothering. They need to find new ways to express themselves which will raise their self-esteem. For this, a counsellor or women's support group is more valuable than a pill.

Women who have interesting jobs, steady incomes, a sense of purpose, or things to do usually report fewer problems with the menopause. Conversely, women without as many options, in unskilled or poorly paid jobs, often view the menopause as more difficult. They may have less information about the physical symptoms of the menopause and react to them with more anxiety. Other unrelated illnesses may exist which compound the problem. The medical profession usually handles health problems with surgery, medicines, or tranquillizers, but frequently doesn't provide the kind of information and counselling that is needed to combat fears and years of negative stereotypes.

Cultural anthropologists who look at women's roles in various societies believe the social context of our lives determines our reactions to ageing. In our culture, the emphasis on youth and the nuclear family structure can make the menopause a lonely time for women. In many other cultures, ageing increases the status, power, and freedom that women experience. Instead of bringing depression, the menopausal years bring recognition and leadership roles in the extended family, ceremonies, and commerce. Freedom from sexual taboos allows women to travel more easily. Post-menopausal women are able to cultivate the more assertive side of their nature. Some of this can be seen in our own society if we look at older women who learn new skills, return to college, go into politics, or excel in their professions. What's expected of us often determines what we will be.

HORMONAL FACTORS

Let's examine the opposite viewpoint, that many psychological problems in the menopause *are* directly related to decreasing oestrogen levels. This is an unpopular stance with feminists, because it presents a picture of a woman as irrational and at the mercy of her hormones. It has also contributed to the widespread prescription of oestrogen, tranquillizers, and antidepressant pills. Is there some validity to the viewpoint that emphasizes the chemistry of our inner environment over our reactions to the outside world?

Depression and anxiety, as well as positive mood states, are currently being studied from a biochemical perspective. The brain produces certain compounds that make us feel contented and euphoric, in response to exercise, food, love, meditation, and other stimuli. Other compounds in the brain can make us irritable and depressed. Some women experience marked mood shifts in relation to their hormonal changes, reporting tension before each menstrual period or depression after having a child. In fact, one in 500 women becomes so depressed after giving birth that she is said to have a postpartum psychosis.

During both menopause and giving birth there is a rapid drop in levels of oestrogen and progesterone. It is possible that this shift may trigger depression in some susceptible people. Studies have been done to evaluate the role of oestrogen replacement (hormone replacement therapy) in the mental and emotional status of menopausal women. While the drug is not helpful with major depressions or psychoses, it has had beneficial effects on the moods of some women with more minor problems. Certain studies have shown that women with menopausal problems feel more cheerful, relaxed, and self-confident, and have improved memory and

69

concentration after taking oestrogen. Proponents of oestrogen replacement feel that negative mental states may be directly caused by the menopause and alleviated by oestrogen. Opponents think any improvement seen with oestrogen is due to the alleviation of hot flushes and night sweats, which secondarily improves mood by promoting sounder sleep and decreased anxiety about hot flushes.

It is difficult to resolve these questions with our present knowledge – there's probably truth in both positions. Our psychology – our moods, our outlook on life – is affected by the world around us *and* by our inner biology. The interactions between all these factors are so intimate that it is artificial to try to separate them. During the menopausal years the body goes through a major transition which is experienced differently by every woman, depending on her general health, her body awareness, and the rate at which her hormone levels drop. Her psychological reaction to this transitional phase will be determined by both her biochemistry and her outer circumstances. Each affects the other – inner and outer worlds are inseparable, and in constant interaction.

Psychologists once proclaimed 'biology is destiny', meaning that women were bound to go through certain predictable physical and emotional stages because of their reproductive systems. A more balanced viewpoint is that biology is only a part of destiny, along with the social environment in which we live. Moreover, as we understand this riddle we can direct at least some of our destiny by choosing to enhance our health and self-esteem.

Women reading this chapter may apply it individually according to their own experiences. Some will be pleased to discover they need not become depressed or 'go crazy' just because their periods stop. They need not experience the 'raging imbalance of hormones' they have heard about. Other readers may feel their emotional symptoms are intimately tied to their menopause, and will find relief in the knowledge that hormones can affect mood and emotions.

Menopausal women with physical or psychological problems are frequently given potent medications instead of the information and counselling they may need. Tranquillizers, sedatives, and antidepressants will only mask the issues, and should be avoided unless their use is really necessary for serious emotional problems. These drugs are often addictive and may have unpleasant side effects. Try counselling, exercise, relaxation techniques, and good nutrition first – the side effects of *these* measures make you feel better, not worse. Sometimes what women need above all is to find or establish a self-help group of other midlife women to develop a more positive image of the menopause and ageing.

Gail had a very hectic job and had got into the habit of taking tranquillizers to calm down. When she went through the

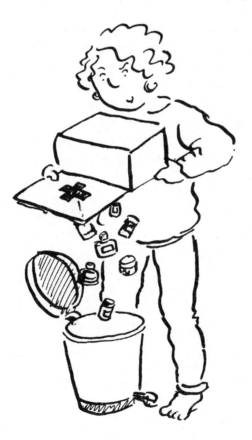

menopause her doctor gave her oestrogen, a progestogen, diuretics and tranquillizers. Later she was given muscle relaxants. She drank a fair amount of coffee throughout the day and alcohol at night to calm down. One day as Gail stood in front of her medicine cabinet she knew something was wrong. She felt terrible inside, shaky and weak. She realized that she never allowed herself to feel the normal state of her body – she was always taking something to alter it. Her medicine cabinet became a blur of yellow, orange, green, and white pills. 'I'm going to stop all these drugs,' she heard herself say. Gail found it very difficult and had to take time off work, but she did manage to stop taking all the pills. She found that acupuncture helped her withdrawal problems, as did joining a self-help group. Now she just has a hectic job, but no drug problem. 'I like knowing what my body is going through,' said Gail. 'I'd rather have a hot flush or an anxious hour than be in a chemical fog.'

Some women may, however, want to try oestrogen replacement for their physical and psychological symptoms. They should read Chapter 10 on the pros and cons of oestrogen replacement (hormone replacement treatment), and evaluate their response to the medicine with understanding and caution.

9.
WHEN PERIODS STOP BEFORE FORTY

Mary's periods became very light and far apart when she was 30. A few years later they disappeared entirely and she began having hot flushes. Mary lived in a remote country area and rarely went to the doctor. When she was in hospital for a broken leg at 36, it was found that she had some osteoporosis, and blood tests revealed she was post-menopausal. Mary's doctor suggested that she take oestrogens, a progestogen at the end of each month, and daily calcium pills. She helped Mary understand the importance of taking these medicines and having yearly check ups. Mary was pleased that her hot flushes went away and she had no more pain with intercourse. She read a good book on the menopause and understood what had happened to her.

Menopause is considered early or premature if it occurs before the age of 40. The most common reason for early menopause is surgical removal of the uterus and ovaries, but occasionally a woman goes into natural menopause before 40. In this chapter we will look at both natural and surgical premature menopause, discuss the problems of this condition, and make recommendations for preserving health and sexuality despite the cessation of periods.

CONDITIONS THAT ARE NOT PREMATURE MENOPAUSE

When a woman in her twenties or thirties stops having menstrual periods there may be many reasons for it. Pregnancy, stress, or illness are common causes, and weight loss, prolonged strenuous exercise, or excessive weight gain can also play a role. Stopping the birth control pill may cause periods to cease for a year or more. Occasionally an excess of prolactin, 'the milk-promoting hormone', interrupts periods and causes milky fluid on the nipples.

Each of these conditions – none of which is premature menopause – needs to be considered when a woman's periods stop prematurely. Blood tests to diagnose premature menopause focus mainly on two hormones that stimulate ovulation. They are called follicle-stimulating hormone (FSH) and luteinizing hormone (LH). When these hormones are low, the ovaries are temporarily at rest, but the woman is not menopausal. The ovaries will generally resume their activity when a woman's general health, emotional well-being, or hormone balance improves – more FSH and LH will be secreted, the ovaries will be stimulated, and ovulation and menstruation will occur.

WHAT IS PREMATURE MENOPAUSE?

Sometimes the levels of FSH and LH are found to be very high. The ovaries are bombarded by stimuli, but do not respond with ovulation, because the areas in the ovaries which produce egg cells are scarce and non-functional. This is premature menopause. There is often a genetic basis for this rare condition – the cells in the ovaries were programmed from birth to function for a shorter time because they were few in number or because of an abnormal gene. Many aspects of this condition are still not completely understood.

When premature menopause occurs in a woman's thirties, she

usually gets hot flushes in the same way older women do. If it occurs even earlier, her symptoms may be less noticeable. Some young women have menstrual periods for only a few years – and they never experience hot flushes. The current explanation is these women have never become accustomed to a high oestrogen level so they do not react to its withdrawal (see Chapter 4).

PREGNANCY AND PREMATURE MENOPAUSE

Premature menopause can be extremely disappointing to the woman who wants to become pregnant. However, some women with a naturally occurring early menopause do conceive after hormone treatment. Those who desire pregnancy should consult a gynaecologist who specializes in infertility problems. In some cases treatment with oestrogen or other medicines, will restore ovulation and fertility, at least for a time.

EARLY MENOPAUSE FROM SURGERY

Though naturally occurring premature menopause is rare, surgically induced early menopause is quite common today, especially in the United States. About 25% of women who have hysterectomies under the age of 40 also have both ovaries removed (if even one ovary is left in, the woman will continue to secrete oestrogen and progesterone and will not experience menopausal symptoms until her late forties or early fifties). Sometimes removing both ovaries is absolutely essential, such as in cases of overwhelming infection, tumours, or cancer.

However, sometimes the ovaries are removed because the gynaecologist has been taught they are not important once the uterus is removed. The argument against this view, and in favour of retaining the ovaries whenever possible, is discussed in Chapter 3. The crucial point requires open discussion with the doctor *before* surgery, so women can make the informed choices.

If a young woman's ovaries are removed in surgery, she will undergo an abrupt premature menopause. She will not have the

75

gradual decrease in oestrogen experienced by women with a natural menopause, so her symptoms may be more intense. Hot flushes can occur immediately after surgery unless oestrogen replacement is started promptly. Most women with this condition decide to take oestrogen tablets to prevent hot flushes and vaginal dryness. Others take oestrogen for a time and then stop it because of side effects, fear of side effects, or the inconvenience of taking a pill daily.

When Carolyn was 25 she developed a severe infection in her tubes and ovaries, possibly associated with an IUD she had been using. Despite hospital treatment and antibiotics it was necessary to remove her uterus and both ovaries in order to control the infection. She was given oestrogen pills to prevent the symptoms of premature menopause. Carolyn was very unhappy and resentful about what had happened to her. At one point a friend persuaded her to stop taking the oestrogen and try multivitamins and herbal capsules, but she developed severe hot flushes and vaginal dryness whenever she did so. Ultimately she resolved to stay on oestrogen until her mid-forties, and then taper the dose a bit. With time and counselling she regained a positive outlook, and pursued a successful career. Later she married and adopted a baby.

What is the best advice for the woman with premature menopause? Should she take replacement hormones? What does she need to know to make a wise decision?

REPLACEMENT HORMONES

Copying nature as closely as possible has many advantages in this situation. The ovaries normally secrete oestrogen and related hormones until the age of 50, and androgens thereafter into old age. Some of these androgens are converted to oestrogen in the body fat (see Chapter 3). The woman with premature menopause can duplicate this situation by taking a moderate dose of oestrogen (hormone replacement therapy) until her mid-forties, a lower dose until the age of 50, and a very small dose or none at all thereafter. This regime will have beneficial effects on her sexual adjustment, although it may not completely restore her sex drive (see Chapter 5). It will also act to prevent osteoporosis (see Chapter 7), which otherwise might begin earlier in life and cause fractures at a younger age.

Women whose ovaries are removed by surgery before their normal menopause run a higher risk of having a heart attack later on. The reason for this is believed to be that the body's oestrogen alters the level and types of blood fats in a healthy way. When the ovaries are removed this protection is missing, but replacement oestrogen in pill form can produce a similar effect, as discussed in Chapter 10.

In deciding to take oestrogen, the woman with premature menopause is helping to prevent discomfort and the long-term problems of heart and bone disease (osteoporosis). At the same time the medication may cause her some problems. No oestrogen taken by mouth can exactly copy the complex ebb and flow of natural hormone secretions. The known side effects from oestrogen replacement are discussed in detail in the following chapter. Although most women with premature menopause do decide to take oestrogen, some do not. For these women it is especially important to guard against osteoporosis and heart disease with exercise and good nutrition. They should exercise vigorously every day to keep their bones strong and promote fitness. They should not smoke or drink excess alcohol. They should eat a very low-fat, high-calcium diet without too much protein, to prevent osteoporosis. They would do well to consult a doctor who is interested in preventive medicine, so they can monitor their levels of blood cholesterol and bone calcium.

These are the problems related to premature menopause, but there's an advantage on the other side of the equation – the risk of breast cancer is lessened! The earlier a woman experiences menopause, the less likely she is to develop breast cancer. Unfortunately, this reduced risk does not necessarily hold true for women on long-term oestrogen replacement treatment (hormone replacement therapy – see Chapter 10).

10.
HORMONE REPLACEMENT THERAPY (HRT)

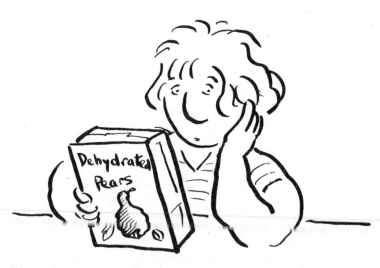

The women in my therapy group were discussing taking oestrogen (hormone replacement therapy or HRT). 'After I talked to my doctor I felt like I'd shrivel up totally if I didn't take it,' said Wendy. 'Then I read an article on vitamin E and ginseng and decided to take those instead.' 'I don't feel I need anything as powerful as oestrogen,' said Roberta. 'I've been thinking about how to stay healthy and it doesn't make sense to keep putting an artificial hormone into my body. Besides, my daughter's always reminding me about all the side effects they've discovered about the pill.' Finally Carol spoke up – 'It's been really important for me to take oestrogen. It's made me feel much better mentally and physically. And I'm so glad to be rid of hot flushes and be able to sleep right through the night.' 'I wish there was a lot more research on this question,' said Clara. 'I'm going to wait until I see better evidence in support of oestrogen, and by then I'll probably be too old to care one way or the other.'

Amazing advances in chemistry and pharmacology in our time have created many new choices for doctors and patients. Common discomforts and ageing itself are no longer accepted as inevitable. Instead they are combatted with medicines and procedures, some very helpful – and others potentially dangerous. We must all tackle the difficult task of choosing reasonably among the possible therapies for our problems. Sometimes just waiting is a good choice, and sometimes treatment is necessary. The menopausal woman's choice about using HRT or not is especially problematic, because the treatment is relatively new, controversial, and unessential, yet quite helpful to some. The benefits and risks of taking oestrogen – and not taking it – vary from person to person. In this chapter we look at the pros, cons, and unknowns of HRT in detail. The following chapter summarizes the information more briefly and provides a self-rating scale to help you make a careful decision, together with your doctor.

A LITTLE HISTORY

Since the beginnings of human evolution, women have gone through the menopause without taking hormones. It's true that surviving at all to middle age was once pretty rare, but for centuries many people have lived to old age, women often outliving men. In places where many women and men live today to be 100 – remote mountainous areas in Ecuador, Pakistan, or southern Russia – the use of HRT is certainly very low! Extreme longevity seems to depend not on any drug therapy, but on a favourable family history and a lifestyle characterized by exercise, moderate eating and drinking, and an optimistic attitude.

When oestrogen was first isolated in the 1920s, it was given to women who had lost their ovaries through surgery, as well as to women with severe problems after a natural menopause. However, its use was not widespread until the 1960s, when oestrogen replacement (HRT) became increasingly popular among middle- and upper-class women in the United States. Women wanted HRT because they were told they would age more slowly, look more attractive, and avoid the discomforts of the menopause. Many doctors promoted HRT because it was a powerful and effective new treatment that provided an apparently quick answer to problems that were hard to deal with, like hot flushes, insomnia, vaginal soreness, midlife crises, and depression. While HRT does deal with the first three problems, it does not necessarily solve the social and psychological difficulties of the middle years. Helping a patient clarify such problems through counselling takes more time than the average doctor can spare, so HRT was a useful substitute.

Another interested party in this use of oestrogen has been the drug companies which manufacture the multitude of pills, injections, and creams designed for menopausal women. In the United States today 30 to 40 million women are post-menopausal, and by 1975, in some middle-class areas, more than half the post-menopausal women used HRT.

In the mid-1970s reports began to appear linking oestrogen use in post-menopausal women to cancer of the uterus. Women were found to be about five times more likely to develop this cancer if they used HRT. There was a rapid decline in the prescription of HRT after these reports, and this decline lasted several years. Recently, however, new studies show that the addition of a progestogen for 10 to 14 days at the end of each 25 day course of oestrogen protects women quite effectively against uterine cancer. As this reassuring news became known, doctors began to prescribe post-menopausal hormones again quite liberally.

It has been said that widespread use of the birth control pill by young women represents an unprecedented socio-medical experiment. Never before in human history has a powerful medicine been taken so widely by healthy people to achieve a goal – contraception – that could be met in other ways. The widespread use of HRT represents a similar experiment. Never before in human history has a large proportion of ageing women taken medicines to prolong the youthful hormonal state of the reproductive years into the fifties and sixties and beyond. This alteration of the natural plan for the human body may have both benefits and risks, which need to be uncovered by painstaking study. Some questions about the effects of HRT are being answered, but some are still being debated. What are the types of oestrogen currently available and what are their advantages and disadvantages?

OESTROGEN – TYPES AND METHODS OF USE

Three types of oestrogen occur naturally – oestrone, oestradiol, and oestriol. Chemical variations of these three forms are used as medicines, and their differing actions and potencies are debated among pharmacologists. Dosage and the method of administration also affect women's responses to particular forms of oestrogen.

Most oestrogen tablets currently on the market are composed of various forms of oestrone or oestradiol. Oestradiol is the principal oestrogen naturally present in women before the menopause and oestrone is the main oestrogen present after the menopause. Oestrone and oestradiol are very similar and each can be converted into the other within the body.

One of the most commonly prescribed forms of oestrogen today is available under the brand name Premarin. It is a mixture of oestrone and other forms of oestrogen. It is popular because it is natural, being derived from pregnant mares' urine, rather than synthesized in the laboratory. However, there is no real evidence for or against the use of natural oestrogens as opposed to the synthetic ones currently on the market, such as Harmogen or oestradiol.

In my opinion, women should not take any oestrogen which is combined with a tranquillizer. Tranquillizers cause sedation and can be habit forming. Experts believe that they should be used only when absolutely necessary for anxiety, and never given with a drug designed for daily administration. Menopausal women should probably avoid taking the so called non-steroidal oestrogens, such as DES (diethylstilboesterol), because of the association of these drugs with vaginal cancer in the female children of women who took the medicines during pregnancy. The non-steroidal oestrogens are chemically less similar to natural oestrogens, and need further safety evaluation. Another form of oestrogen to be avoided is the injectable type, which in one study was associated with a higher risk of breast cancer.

Oestrogen is also available in adhesive patches which are applied to the skin of the abdomen or thigh. The hormone is gradually and evenly absorbed through the skin over a $3\frac{1}{2}$ day period. The patches are changed twice a week, but the woman is free to bathe or swim at any time. There may be significant advantages and disadvantages to using oestrogen by skin patch compared to the usual tablet form. When oestrogen is taken by tablet it is absorbed through the intestinal tract and travels immediately to the liver, where it stimulates the production of a substance which causes high blood pressure in some individuals. Since oestrogen by skin patch avoids this step it seems to be preferable for women prone to blood pressure problems. On the other hand, there is concern that oestrogen absorbed through the skin may not have the same favourable effect on blood cholesterol that is found with oral tablets. More study is needed on these questions.

USE OF A PROGESTOGEN WITH OESTROGEN

Oestrogen used alone after the menopause has been associated with an increased risk of cancer of the uterus. This risk can be greatly reduced or eliminated by adding a progestogen tablet daily in the last 10 to 14 days of the cycle. Progestogens are compounds similar to progesterone, normally secreted by the ovaries after ovulation and in pregnancy. Natural progesterone is less effective when taken orally, but progestogens can be taken in tablet form. It is extremely important for any woman who still has her uterus to use the following kind of schedule if she wishes to take oestrogen. She should take an oestrogen pill from the first to the twenty-fifth day of the month, and should also take a progestogen tablet from the fourteenth to the twenty-fifth day. Then she should stop taking both tablets for five or six days, and at this point she will usually have some bleeding. The progestogen tablet has the effect of allowing the lining of the uterus to be evenly shed when all the hormones are stopped. If the lining is sloughed off this way every month, it is highly unlikely that it will become cancerous.

If a woman's uterus has been removed by surgery, she should take a few days off oestrogen each month, but she need not take a progestogen. Any woman who has a uterus, however, should take a progestogen whenever she takes daily oestrogen. The addition of a progestogen is also a good idea for a woman who has taken oestrogen alone in the past and is no longer taking it. A ten day course of a progestogen will help her get rid of any excess uterus lining that might have built up. Some doctors prescribe a progestogen even if oestrogen has never been taken, especially in women who seem to produce abundant natural oestrogen after the menopause. This occurs more often in women who have considerable body fat.

The right amount of progestogen to take is the smallest possible effective dose. Recent studies indicate that a lower dose than the one usually prescribed today is effective for most post-menopausal women. Women should consult their doctors on the details of this question, and pharmaceutical companies should provide tablets in convenient low doses.

Adding progestogen to the oestrogen cycle greatly reduces the risk of cancer of the uterus, but it also has disadvantages. Progestogen compounds in the birth control pill were found to cause changes in the body's use of starches and sugars similar to the changes of diabetes, and to alter blood fats in an unfavourable way. They were implicated, along with oestrogen, in high blood pressure, heart disease, and strokes. These risks may be greater than the danger of cancer of the uterus. This kind of comparison needs to be made individually for each woman, based on her personal and family medical history.

Progestogens currently on the market include Depo-Provera, Provera, Minovlar, and Gynovlar. Research is needed to clarify the differences among these compounds in terms of side effects and to determine the lowest effective dose.

REASONS FOR TAKING POST-MENOPAUSAL OESTROGENS

Let us review the reasons women and their doctors favour using oestrogens, and the dosages appropriate in each situation. Women under the age of 45 who have had a surgical menopause should read Chapter 9 again before reading this section:

Hot Flushes: Oestrogen will act rapidly to reduce this problem. The lowest dose that will prevent discomfort is the goal, and therefore women should keep a record of their hot flushes and start with the lowest dose of oestrogen available.

Oestrogen tablets are usually quickly effective in reducing the distress from hot flushes. However, the symptom generally returns when oestrogen is stopped. Taking oestrogen, therefore, does not cure hot flushes but it does postpone them until the time that HRT is stopped. Some women elect to take oestrogen indefinitely and thus may never have hot flushes. Other women take oestrogen for temporary relief of hot flushes and then decide to stop it after a few months or a few years. Since the reasons for hot flushes are related to rapid decrease in natural oestrogen levels (see Chapter 4), the best way to cease HRT is to taper it off very slowly. The woman taking .625 mg of oestrogen daily can switch to .3 mg daily for a month or two, then take this dose every other day, and finally stop it entirely. She should continue with a progestogen in the second half of each cycle unless her uterus has been removed. Sometimes after a three to six month trial of this regime, hot flushes will be lessened. If not, the woman can resume taking oestrogen and repeat the tapering off process when she is ready. Many women find they can cope with the problem of hot flushes when they gradually and slowly reduce the oestrogen dose this way.

If oestrogen cannot be used, some doctors use injectable or oral progestogens alone to relieve hot flushes. These medications are not as effective as oestrogen, but do help in some cases. However, they do have side effects of their own, particularly irregular bleeding.

Vaginal Soreness: Insertion of the penis, fingers, or a vaginal speculum can be uncomfortable or painful in post-menopausal women, because oestrogen and androgen secretion from the ovaries has decreased. One action of these hormones is to keep the vaginal lining cells thickened and resistant to friction. When hormone levels drop, this cellular layer becomes thinner, drier, and less elastic. The vagina is then more likely to be sore or irritated by penetration. This situation can be alleviated by taking oestrogen tablets, or by the use of a low-dose oestrogen cream. Some women, who do not want to take oestrogen orally, use a hormonal cream very successfully.

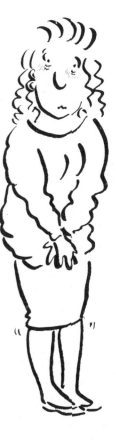

If a woman is taking oral oestrogen, even in the smallest doses, she will generally not need to use vaginal oestrogen creams. The low-dose cream treatment advocated in this section is designed for women who want to alleviate vaginal soreness without taking other forms of oestrogen.

One of the commonly used oestrogen creams is Premarin cream, which comes with an applicator calibrated for 1 g to 4 g cream. The dose frequently suggested is 2 g to 4 g daily (a half to one applicator full) applied vaginally. As there is .625 mg of Premarin per gram of the cream, this dose would give a woman 1.25 to 2.5 mg of oestrogen daily. However, lower doses of oestrogen cream than currently suggested by most doctors and drug companies are effective. A recent British study showed that vaginal soreness responds to as little as .1 mg of oestrogen daily in cream form. The oestrogen is rapidly absorbed from the vagina. In fact, oestrogen cream can be stronger than pills, as hormones from the cream enter the blood stream directly and are not subject to the digestive process.

The cream should be directed towards the sore area which is usually inside the inner vaginal lips right at the entrance to the vagina. Apply the cream to that area with the applicator or with a finger, being sure to get to the sorest point. After five to ten days of such treatment, the problem of pain with penetration is usually resolved. Thereafter, most women then use the cream every two or three days. Do not use the cream just before intercourse – it is designed for vaginal treatment, and not as a lubricant.

One study suggested that after about a week of oestrogen cream use with these very low doses, the vaginal cells seem to erect a partial barrier to the systemic absorption of oestrogens, so no increased blood levels of oestrogen were found. However, more research is needed to clarify the effects of the very low doses of cream required to relieve vaginal discomfort.

Other oestrogen creams besides Premarin may be used, following the same suggestions for lower dosage. Most are effective after a week of daily use of only a very small amount of cream.

When such small doses are used, is there a risk of cancer of the uterus? Probably not, but to be safe, some doctors recommend the use of a progestogen for ten days after a few months of cream use, and every six months thereafter.

The use of these minimal doses of oestrogen cream eliminates most of the pain of vaginal penetration. However, it does not restore as much vaginal lubrication as was present before the menopause, so it is wise to use an oil or cream for lubrication during intercourse.

Androgen cream (a water-soluble cream containing 1% to 2% of the hormone testosterone) is also effective in preventing vaginal soreness after the menopause. It is used in the same way as oestrogen cream. After a week or so of daily application, minimal amounts are effective twice weekly. No studies have been published that compare the use of oestrogen and androgen creams.

Osteoporosis (Brittle Bones): As Chapter 7 spells out, HRT retards the loss of calcium from the bones after the menopause. Since HRT results in a lower rate of hip and forearm fractures and height loss, doctors often suggest that women most at risk of osteoporosis begin HRT after the menopause and continue it for the rest of their lives. If HRT is stopped at any point, the bones rapidly lose any beneficial effects.

We don't know the exact dose of oestrogen needed to prevent bone fractures. Probably protection increases with increasing dosages, but some benefit is derived even from small amounts. Healthy living, including daily walks and other exercise and an increased calcium intake, as detailed in Chapter 7, will also help promote stronger bones.

WHAT HRT WON'T DO

Though HRT has been shown to be helpful with hot flushes, vaginal soreness, and osteoporosis, it has *not* been proved to be helpful in preventing wrinkles or other signs of ageing, or in treating urinary incontinence or psychological problems. The effect of HRT on the heart and circulation are variable and complex – some studies show a protective effect, and others show increased risk. The results of these studies are summarized later in this chapter.

HRT is not designed to correct hormonal imbalances in menstruating women. It should generally not be taken until periods have stopped completely, because while they continue, the ovaries are producing natural oestrogen. Before the menopause a progestogen sometimes helps regulate bleeding problems.

REASONS FOR NOT TAKING POST-MENOPAUSAL OESTROGENS

Cancer Of The Uterus: The main reason many women stopped HRT after 1975 was the finding that the medication increased the risk of developing cancer of the uterus. Fortunately, the cancers occurring in 95% of these women responded well to hysterectomy and other treatments. Subsequently it has been found that the use of a progestogen in the second half of each oestrogen cycle allows for complete shedding of the lining of the uterus and very substantially reduces the risk of cancer of the uterus. Some studies suggest that the risk of uterine cancer is even lower among oestrogen and progestogen users than among women who have never used HRT. The cancer risk remains, however, because some doctors do not prescribe a progestogen for an adequate time each month (10 to 14 days) and some women neglect to take it.

Obesity also increases the risk of cancer of the uterus, because of the increased amount of natural oestrogen formed in the body's fat cells. Menopausal women who are more than 25 or 30 pounds overweight are not advised to take oestrogen in most cases. They should take a ten day course of a progestogen to promote a shedding of the uterus lining, which protects against this type of cancer. If bleeding occurs, some doctors suggest that they repeat the progestogen every few months until there is no further bleeding.

Liver And Gall Bladder Disease: As a rare complication, taking oestrogen can induce liver tumours. It is therefore wise for doctors to check for liver enlargement in women using HRT. Women with liver disease due to alcohol or other causes should take no unnecessary medications, including oestrogen.

Women taking oestrogen have been found to have an increased risk of gall bladder disease in several studies. They require surgical removal of the gall bladder more than twice as often as other women. The women most at risk of gallstones are those who are obese, have a high cholesterol dietary intake or blood level, or have diabetes, Crohn's disease, or some other rare illnesses. Any woman who has these risks or knows she has gallstones should avoid HRT, and should consume foods high in fibre (whole grains, beans, and vegetables) and very low in fat. Most people can avoid gall bladder surgery this way.

Depression: While some post-menopausal women have found that oestrogen improves their mood, others find they are depressed by it, or by the added progestogen. Such depression is sometimes related to an increased need for B vitamins and improved by the daily use of vitamin B-complex pill containing 25 mg of vitamin B_6.

If depression persists unrelated to any obvious factors in daily life, women can stop HRT to assess differences in their moods.

Uterine Fibroids: Uterine fibroids are benign overgrowths of muscular tissue (tumours), which enlarge the uterus. They are stimulated by oestrogen. Ordinarily any fibroid tumours present shrink after the menopause, because of decreased oestrogen levels and are rarely any further problem. However, HRT may cause continued growth of these tumours. Sometimes fibroids grow to a size that is uncomfortable and a hysterectomy is suggested. It is safer and easier to avoid HRT if fibroids are growing.

More Visits To The Doctor: Women who take oestrogen generally visit their doctor more frequently for routine check-ups. It is a good idea for them to have a blood pressure and breast examination twice a year and an overall physical examination with blood chemistry tests yearly. If they experience any vaginal bleeding at times other than the five days they are off the pills they should have a biopsy or a D and C to test the uterus lining.

These are recommendations for more medical care than is usual for post-menopausal women. Ideally, older women should visit a doctor once a year for an examination and screening tests, but many fail to do so after their reproductive years and seek care only for illness. On the one hand, more frequent visits may result in earlier recognition of abnormalities. On the other hand, they are time consuming, and result in more medical tests and drugs, some of which may be harmful.

Daily Pill Taking And Monthly Periods: Many people dislike taking pills regularly. Women using HRT to prevent osteoporosis are advised to continue it for the rest of their lives, but they may become bored or forgetful with this regime. Others dislike it they had expected freedom from them.

CONTROVERSIES OVER HRT

The two areas where HRT is most controversial today are

cardiovascular disease and breast cancer. Some research claims that HRT causes or worsens these conditions, while other studies show no effects or even benefits. When controversy prevails, it usually means the answers are complex and the right questions may not yet have been asked. Here's the currently available evidence:

Heart Attacks, Strokes, And High Blood Pressure: Since heart disease is the leading cause of death in older women, it is important to know the effects of HRT on the heart and blood vessels. However, at present the evidence is contradictory, with some studies showing a reduction in risk for high blood pressure and heart attack when women use HRT and others showing the opposite. Part of the confusion may stem from the fact that most studies have involved women on different types and dosages of oestrogen, to which a week or two of progestogen may or may not have been added. Experts in this field are currently saying that oestrogen alone, in low doses, may provide some protection against heart disease. Oestrogen use results in lower levels of total blood cholesterol and somewhat higher amounts of a type of cholesterol that seems to protect against blood vessel damage. However, the progestogen added to oestrogen at the end of each month is believed to act in the other direction, increasing the risk of blood vessel damage, stroke, and heart attack, by altering the type of fats in the blood stream in an unfavourable way.

It is ironic that progestogen, so effective in preventing cancer of the uterus, may ultimately have a negative effect on the circulatory system. Women who have had a hysterectomy and therefore do not need added progestogen may derive some protection from heart disease by using HRT. But women who must use an added progestogen may ultimately run an increased risk of heart and blood vessel disease. The extent of this possible negative effect and the people at greatest risk are not known. In general the chances of heart disease are greatest in smokers, women with high blood pressure or high cholesterol, diabetes, the very obese, and people who do not exercise. Your doctor can help you assess your own situation.

The effects of HRT on high blood pressure and stroke are similarly confusing at present. While the birth control pill in younger women has been shown to cause high blood pressure in some, this has not been a notable effect of HRT in post-menopausal women. But be cautious. Women taking oestrogen should have blood pressure checks every six months and stop hormones if the pressure rises significantly. If severe headaches develop while taking oestrogen, or if a woman notices any unusual symptoms, such as blurred vision, weakness, or numbness of any part of the body, or unusual pains in the chest or other area, she should stop her pills and seek medical attention.

All women using HRT, with or without progestogen should have periodic checks of their blood glucose and cholesterol levels. Everyone over 50 can diminish the risk of heart disease by following a lifestyle with lots of exercise and a low-fat, low-salt diet, as discussed in Chapters 14 and 15.

Cancer Of The Breast: Studies aimed at determining whether HRT changes the risk of breast cancer have been conflicting. Several studies show an increased risk after long-term use, especially in women who develop benign breast lumps after beginning HRT. Other studies fail to show such risks. There is also controversy about whether women with intact ovaries are at greater or lesser risk than women whose ovaries have been surgically removed. We do know that women with a surgical menopause have less chance of developing breast cancer if they do *not* use HRT. If they do use it, their risk of breast cancer appears to rise to approximately that of women with intact ovaries.

Overall, many researchers feel that there is a slight association between the use of HRT and the subsequent development of breast cancer. This means that HRT is by no means the only factor involved in the onset of breast cancer, but may be a promoting factor in some women. The risk appears to rise with the dose of hormones used and the length of time they are taken. Other risk factors for breast cancer are the presence of benign breast lumps with atypical cells, a family history of breast cancer, and not having borne children.

In addition, several dietary factors have been implicated in breast cancer, such as a high content of fat, protein, or overall calories in the diet, and the use of alcohol. Recent studies have shown a possible connection between even moderate alcohol use (three drinks a week) and breast cancer, with increased risks for heavier drinkers. See Chapter 15 for more details.

At present our knowledge in this area is incomplete, which leaves women and their doctors in a dilemma. It is wise for most women to use HRT in the lowest possible dose if they do decide to take it. Women should do breast self-examinations monthly, be checked by a doctor every six months, and stop HRT if breast lumps develop, even if they are benign. Women with existing benign breast lumps that have atypical cells may be at greater risk of developing cancer later and should probably avoid HRT altogether. Mammography (x-rays of breast tissue) should be performed every year or two as needed, depending on the woman's family history and personal risk factors. Safe new techniques of visualizing body tissue, such as nuclear magnetic resonance (NMR), may also prove helpful in the detection of breast cancer.

Breast cancer is justifiably a major worry among midlife women. It is important for all women to examine their breasts regularly and to seek medical care promptly if a breast lump is discovered. It is helpful to do breast examinations lying down in bed at night or in the bath. Remember that most lumps are *not* cancer but all should be professionally evaluated. A caffeine-free diet may decrease breast lumpiness, and a low-fat, high-fibre diet may reduce the risk of breast cancer. Suggestions for these changes are given in Chapter 14. If a cancer is found it is important to consider all the options for treatment. Consult with a doctor or cancer specialist who keeps up-to-date with medical research and read all you can find on the subject.

11.
SHOULD YOU HAVE HRT?

After carefully considering the pros and cons of HRT and consulting her doctor, each woman must make a personal decision. Some will want to try HRT to alleviate hot flushes, or may be advised by their doctors to use HRT to prevent osteoporosis or counter premature menopause. Others will know immediately that they do not want to use HRT or may have the health problems listed below that make it unwise for them to use it in any case:

> **Women with these problems should avoid HRT:**
> Cancer of the breast or uterus
> Heart disease, especially if chest pain is present
> Serious high blood pressure
> A history of blood clots in the veins or lungs
> A history of stroke
> Diabetes
> Serious migraine headaches
> Liver disease
> Gallstones or gall bladder disease
> Large uterine fibroids

In addition, women who smoke have a higher risk of heart and circulatory disease, and should not use HRT unless absolutely necessary.

You may want to consider using the following rating system to help you clarify your choice.

THE DECISION TO USE HRT – A PERSONAL RATING SCALE

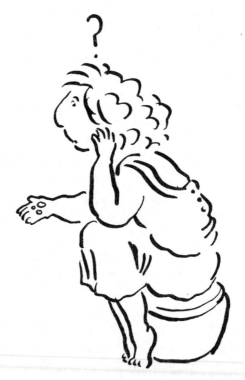

This rating scale is designed to help you clarify your thoughts on whether to use HRT based on your own needs and your personal and family medical history. If you have had your ovaries removed by surgery at any age, you should give a high priority to HRT because you lack the ovarian hormones it will replace. If you are under 45 with a premature menopause, you should generally take hormones until the age of 45 or 50, when you can use this rating scale to decide whether to continue or not.

Since the risk of cancer of the uterus from oestrogen use is virtually eliminated if progestogens are added (see Chapter 10), this risk is not listed as a factor in the scale.

How To Use The Scale: The table on page 95 lists the advantages and disadvantages of HRT. Each has been explained more fully earlier in the book, and is summarized in the pages which follow. Read over each summary section, and then give a score from 0 to 3 to each item on the scale.

When you have given a score to each item, look at the table for some time and think about it. You need not compare your total scores for advantages and disadvantages. The table is not designed to give you a numerical score, but to summarize the data and let you judge how strongly you feel about the benefits and risks of HRT as they are currently known.

Be sure to discuss your questions and conclusions with your doctor, both now and as your knowledge increases and your feelings change. Remember that many women have tried oestrogen and then stopped it – your decision does not have to be final. Remember also the alternative treatments for menopausal problems discussed in this book.

ADVANTAGES OF HRT

Elimination Of Hot Flushes: As discussed in Chapter 4, the use of oestrogen tablets is very effective against hot flushes. However, hot flushes will return if oestrogen is stopped. Slow reduction of your dose can lessen but not eliminate this problem. Alternative methods to deal with hot flushes are discussed in Chapter 4. Give yourself a score of 0 to 3 depending on the importance of this symptom to you.

PERSONAL RATING SCALE – TO DECIDE ON USING HORMONE REPLACEMENT THERAPY OR NOT

Advantages	Score
Elimination of hot flushes	
Elimination of vaginal soreness	
Reduced risk of brittle bones	
Possible decreased risk of heart disease	
Other personal advantages _____	

Disadvantages	Score
Possible increased risk of heart disease or stroke	
Possible increased risk of breast cancer	
Possible increased risk of gall bladder disease	
Possible growth of uterine fibroids	
More medical visits	
Monthly periods continue	
Other personal disadvantages _____	

Scores

0 = not important
1 = little importance
2 = quite important
3 = very important

Remember to read the text before giving a score.

Elimination Of Vaginal Soreness: Oestrogen is very effective in eliminating vaginal soreness due to penetration. However, minimal amounts of vaginal oestrogen cream also do this, as discussed in Chapter 10. If vaginal soreness is the only symptom you want to treat, you can use very small amounts of cream twice weekly and not take oestrogen pills. In this case give yourself a 0 score. If you don't have pain with vaginal penetration, give yourself a 0 score. On the other hand, if oestrogen creams are not satisfactory and you are considering oestrogen pills, rate this item with a score from 0 to 3 depending on its importance to you.

Reduced Risk Of Brittle Bones: As discussed in Chapter 7, oestrogen reduces the risk of brittle bones (osteoporosis) and fractures. To help you decide on the importance of this problem to you, look back to the table of factors that increase the risk of osteoporosis on page 55. Note that the most important risk factors are at the top of both lists and the least important are below the line. You should also know that experts in the field of osteoporosis do not currently agree on the importance of all these factors. There is much more to be learned about what causes and prevents osteoporosis in different people. Therefore, the score you give yourself based on this table will reflect an approximate idea of your risk of osteoporosis, not a precise one.

Tick any items that apply to you on this table. If you have two or more ticks on the *Genetic or Medical Factors* list, you should consider yourself at risk of developing osteoporosis. If you have no ticks on the *Lifestyle Factors* list your risk is lowered, but if you have one or more ticks on this list your risk is increased – unless, of course, you decide to change your habits! If you are thin, especially if you are a thin smoker, your risk of osteoporosis with fractures is high. If you are black, you can consider that you are more protected from osteoporosis than other women, but you should pay attention nonetheless to the factors on the table. Based on your study of this table, give yourself an overall score for the advantage of oestrogen in decreasing brittle bones. If you have made no ticks on either list of the osteoporosis table, give yourself a 0 score. If you have ticked one or more risk factors, give yourself a score of 1 to 3. This item is a difficult one. Think it over and consult with your doctor if possible. Perhaps read Chapter 7 again to help clarify the issues involved.

Possible Decreased Risk Of Heart Disease: The effects of oestrogen on the development of heart disease are not entirely known. Several studies show that low-dose post-menopausal oestrogens protect against heart attacks. If your uterus has been removed, so that you can take oestrogen without an added progestogen, you may lower your risk of heart disease by using HRT. Be sure your blood pressure is not high and does not rise with the use of HRT.

If your uterus is not removed, you must take a progestogen for at least ten days of each month along with oestrogen to prevent cancer of the uterus. This may change or reverse the protective effect of oestrogen on heart disease, as explained in the previous chapter.

Consult your doctor about this question, as it is confusing. Hopefully new research findings will be forthcoming.

Rating this advantage of HRT will depend on whether your uterus has been removed or not. If you have had a hysterectomy, give yourself a score of 0 to 3, depending on the importance to you of a decreased risk of heart disease, based on your personal and family history. If you have a uterus and must therefore use a progestogen, give yourself a 0 score on this item.

Other Personal Advantages: Rate the importance of any other advantages of HRT that you may be aware of. Some women find that it increases their sex drive, helps reduce forgetfulness, or improves their mood. Since these effects are individual, you may need to try HRT to determine its effects on you. Give yourself a 0 to 3 score on each factor that is important to you.

DISADVANTAGES OF HRT

Possible Increased Risk Of Heart Disease Or Stroke: When a progestogen is added to oestrogen to protect against cancer of the uterus, it may increase the risk of heart disease or a stroke. Progestogens change the type of fats in the blood stream, and make it more likely that damage to blood vessels may ultimately occur. Women who have not had a hysterectomy must use a progestogen at the end of each month of oestrogen pills. Until more is known, those with a known risk of heart disease should proceed with caution. Such risks include smoking, high blood pressure, elevated cholesterol level, diabetes, significant obesity, inactivity, and a close family history of heart attacks or strokes. Consult your doctor about these questions. If you have had a hysterectomy (and thus need not use progestogen), give yourself a 0 score on this item. If your uterus is intact, rate the risk with a score from 0 to 3, depending on the importance of this factor to you.

Possible Increased Risk Of Breast Cancer: The effects of HRT on the development of breast cancer are controversial. Several studies have shown a small increased risk after long-term oestrogen use, especially in women who already have benign breast lumps with atypical cells. Other studies have not shown this association. Until more is known, women with a high risk of breast cancer based on family history, not having borne children, or having benign breast lumps should proceed with caution. Consult your doctor about your risk in this area.

Give yourself a score of 0 to 3 based on your personal appraisal of these factors.

Possible Increased Risk Of Gall Bladder Disease: Several studies have shown that gallstones, gall bladder pain, and the necessity for surgical removal of the gall bladder occur more frequently with oestrogen use. Women most at risk of developing gallstones are those who suffer from obesity, high cholesterol levels in the blood, diabetes, Crohn's disease, and some other rare illnesses. A high fibre diet protects against gall bladder disease.

Give yourself a score of 0 to 3 based on your appraisal of your risks.

Possible Growth Of Uterine Fibroids: Oestrogen can cause uterine fibroid tumours to grow larger. While these benign tumours usually shrink after the menopause, they can remain large or continue to grow when oestrogen is taken. If you do not have fibroids, you can give this item a 0 score. If your doctor has told you that you have fibroids of any significant size, discuss this question with him or her, and give yourself a score between 1 and 3.

More Medical Visits: Women who use post-menopausal hormones such as oestrogen, need check ups every 6 to 12 months. Give yourself a score of 0 to 3 based on your feelings about this.

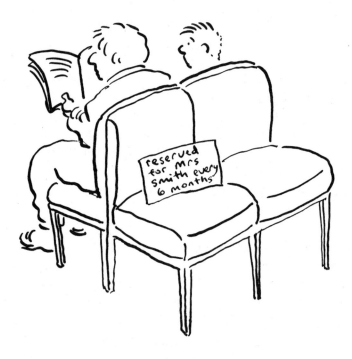

Monthly Periods Continue: When oestrogen with an added progestogen is taken after the menopause, a monthly flow continues, necessitating the use of pads or tampons. This flow rarely causes serious cramps.

Give yourself a score from 0 to 3 depending on your feelings about this. Some women may welcome this menstrual flow and put the score in the advantage column.

Other Personal Disadvantages: Rate the importance to you of any other disadvantage of oestrogen treatment that applies to you. Some women find it difficult to remember to take daily pills, do not like the way they feel on HRT, or think that such a use of hormones is against nature's plan for their bodies. Rate your personal appraisal of these disadvantages from 0 to 3.

12.
POST-
MENOPAUSAL
ZEST

I'm not exactly sure what lies ahead for me . . . this new young woman. It's a brand new role for me. All this freedom to be myself at long last. To really be myself – not what somebody else says I should be or what somebody else expects me to be. I don't know what is around the corner, but I do know that I'm on the path that is taking me there. My feet are willing and light, my spirit is free, and I am feeling wonderful!

As menstrual periods stop, women enter a time in their lives which can be vital and new. Margaret Mead, the well-known anthropologist with an interest in women's roles, coined the term 'post-menopausal zest' for this period.

What is this state? Zest is a quality that gives our lives relish, stimulation, and keen enjoyment. How do we find and keep a sense of zest for living in midlife? Everyone knows some older people who have it – who are vital and involved in the world around them. We also know people of the same age who are depressed, ailing, or reclusive. In this and the following chapters we will consider attitudes to ageing and ways to find and keep a zestful outlook in the second half of life. Some of these concepts have been touched on earlier in this book in relation to special problems of the menopause; but most of the ways to keep zestful are as useful to men as to women.

BELIEFS ABOUT AGEING

Janet was very involved in running her farm, and at 55 she was attending evening classes to learn more about new farming methods. Her husband had died of a sudden heart attack when she was 48. Both her daughters had gone to the city to work. At first she was overwhelmed and thought of selling the farm, but gradually she began to see that she could handle it herself with some new techniques, different cash crops, and the help of a young couple who came to live with her. She realized that she came from a long line of strong farming women. She enjoyed the challenges of outdoor work and farm management, and found she could do many of the things she previously left to her husband. When people admired her work she was fond of saying, 'These past few years have certainly taught this old dog some new tricks.'

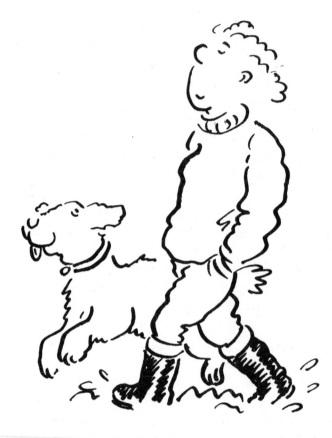

Rebecca lost her job as a secretary after twenty years when her firm went bankrupt. She was 52, and lived alone. She managed to find occasional jobs through a temporary agency but felt financially and emotionally insecure. She called her son on the phone daily and wanted to move in with him, but he had a wife and small child and did not welcome the idea, although he did send her some money every month. Rebecca increased her daily dose of oestrogen and took antidepressants, but she still felt terrible.

She saw no future for herself. She felt she had alienated most of her old friends by refusing to go out with them or crying so easily. At the mental health clinic they suggested she go into hospital and consider shock treatment, but she was frightened by this idea. Rebecca remained depressed, often contemplating suicide but being restrained by her religious beliefs and her attachment to her son and grandchild. After a few years, she slowly began to improve. A friend gave her some back copies of a healthcare magazine, and she started taking vitamins and eating healthier food. She felt a little better, but still had trouble seeing herself as valuable or important in any way. Besides her son and her part-time jobs, she had very few connections to the world around her. She didn't see how she could possibly start any new activities or get any new interests at this stage in her life.

Janet and Rebecca responded very differently to sudden, unexpected change in midlife, but both show how much we are subtly but profoundly influenced by the beliefs about ageing held in our culture. Often our view of other women or ourselves in the menopausal years is a composite of how we saw our own mothers and other family members, and what we glean from the media. Many women have negative memories of their own mothers' menopausal symptoms and a strong dread of ageing. Others have positive, powerful, or serene role models in their families.

It is worth spending some time understanding what your own inner views of the menopause and ageing may be. Close your eyes and picture a woman of 50, in her menopausal years. What does she look like, how does she feel, and how does she move and speak? Write down three adjectives to describe this woman. Do the same for a woman of 60, and then one of 70. Visualize them in your imagination, and then describe each with three adjectives. Look over what you have written, and get an idea of your own fantasies and beliefs about ageing. Do you like these women? Do you want to be like them as you age? If not, what do you want to be like when you are 50, 60, and 70?

Play the game again, and visualize *yourself* at each of those ages. Write down three adjectives to describe yourself at 50, 60, and 70 the way you really want to be. Now look at your two lists. Is your second list – with your personal ideals – different from your first list? What this exercise can do is show you that you don't have to be like your imaginary picture of an older woman if you don't want to be. You can be your unique self, growing older in your own fashion.

Although our culture may have a stereotyped view of men and women at various ages, projected in television, films, and advertisements, real people are incredibly diverse. We are usually happier if we value our uniqueness and do not try to make ourselves fit into the cultural mould. Women who do not accept the prevalent belief that their worth as females depends on youthful sex appeal can value wisdom and strength in middle age. However, if you listen to messages like, 'You can't teach an old dog new tricks', or 'You can't learn new skills after the age of 15 or 25', you will make these prophecies come true for yourself.

To break away from negative beliefs, it helps to find friends who are excited about life after 50 and talk to them about their outlooks, activities, and plans. Gradually you will see a more positive view of human potential in ageing which you can incorporate into your consciousness. Let your fantasy and imagination dwell on these new role models instead of the negative stereotypes the media offer. Think of Margaret Mead or Golda Meir instead of a nagging wife in curlers. Why not?

STAY CONNECTED TO THE WORLD AROUND YOU

Numerous studies of ageing have shown that people connected to a network of others are happier and live longer. While spending time alone is important for quiet self-renewal and creativity, it can be a problem for depressed people who spend it watching television or drinking. Connections to the natural world are also important – animals, plants, walks in the park, and hikes in the countryside. These activities keep us aware of the web of life and help to combat depression.

Community involvement can be important in the second half

of life. We need to use our experience to help direct the larger society in which we live, in whatever way seems most appropriate. Voting is important, but many people can give more than a vote to a cause or organization they believe in. Such individual efforts are the lifeblood of our democratic society, and can give great meaning to those who participate in them.

Middle-aged people who believe in their abilities to keep learning and giving are doing many things in our society. They are returning to college, sometimes finishing a degree at 60 or 70 that they couldn't pursue in their twenties. They are involved in community affairs, politics, or crafts, in addition to holding down jobs. Sometimes they are finding new ways to earn income from their interests. Women who have been mothers, in particular, must redefine themselves in midlife when the parental role has ended. This is important as a bridge to the future, to keep life vital into old age.

One of our important life jobs is to keep discovering and growing until we die. As one wise woman puts it, we must uncover our inner design. This means discovering who we are – amid or beyond our many roles as worker, parent, spouse, or lover – and what really gives our lives meaning. What excites us and makes us grow? What can we best give to the world around us? Such answers are obvious to some people but hard for others to find. Answers vary at different times in our lives. Getting even a partial answer to these questions is energizing. Knowing where you are going in life is an important part of post-menopausal zest.

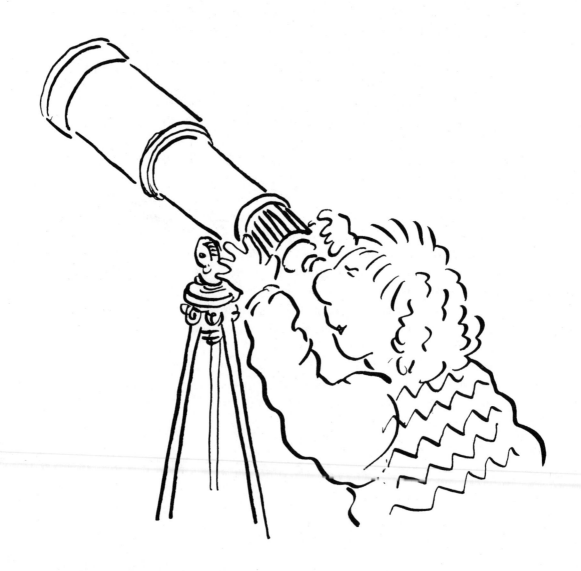

13.
RELAXATION
– CALMING
DOWN AND
LETTING GO

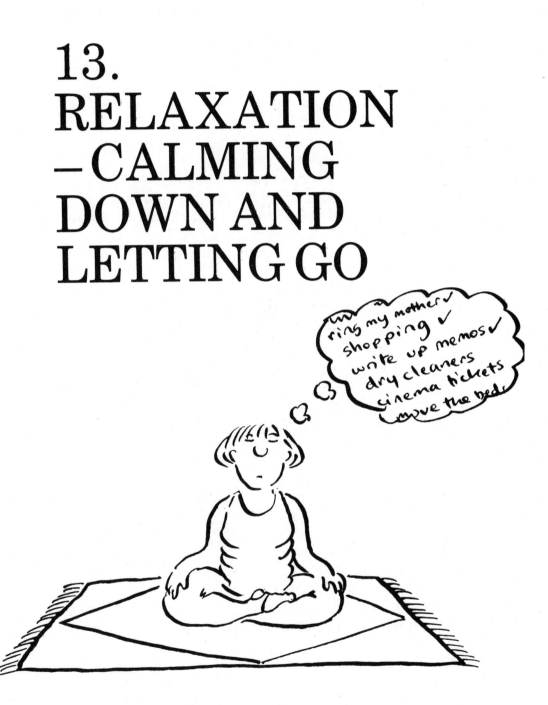

Life is constantly challenging, both physically and psychologically – and cannot be otherwise. Our innate urges to survive, relate to others, learn, and master our environment cause change and conflict. The idea that life can be lived without stress, or that happiness is found in perpetual relaxation is a common misinterpretation of the aims of stress reduction techniques. It has been aptly named 'the Elysian Fields fallacy'.

What we need is the ability to alternate between being alert and energetic on the one hand, and relaxed and calm on the other. This sounds obvious, but many people have difficulty letting go of the tension they accumulate during the day. They are perpetually switched 'on' and can only turn themselves 'off' with alcohol, tranquillizers, or exhaustion and fitful sleep. Some of the reasons for this are obvious. Urban living is crowded, noisy, mechanized, and rushed. The media bombards people with sounds of urgency and scenes of violence or disaster. Competition and 'hurry sickness' are an important part of our culture. 'Hurry sickness' is a term that refers to pervasive feelings of urgency and time pressure, which may contribute to heart disease and other common illnesses of contemporary life.

It is overly simplistic to say that heart disease, cancer, allergies, or ulcers are 'caused' by excessive stress alone. There are many other genetic, environmental, and lifestyle factors involved in these illnesses. However, we can say that many illnesses are aggravated by prolonged, excessive tension – whether it stems from noise, rush, and overwork, or from fear, anger, and self-blame. Conversely, sick people often recover faster, with less pain and disability, when they learn to get rid of excessive tension. Animal research shows that stress or fear depress the immune system, making the body more vulnerable to infections or cancer.

Let's consider some of the factors in everyday life which can be changed to lower tension and restore balance to our nervous systems.

Noise is an obvious place to start. Many people are constantly bombarded by noise, which causes tension, fatigue, and high blood pressure. Noise at work and in cities may be unavoidable, but noise at home can be minimized. Anyone who feels overstressed should experiment with turning off the television, radio, and loud music, and living with silence. Even short periods of silence during the day are helpful to enable our nervous systems to rebalance. In the Quaker tradition, silence is used for worship and for the beginning and end of business meetings and ceremonies. It enables the participants to renew themselves, hear their inner spirits, and go forth to be effective in dealing with the problems of the world.

Many people repeatedly drink coffee or tea during the day, giving themselves a caffeine 'high' that comes from stimulation of the adrenal glands and the central nervous system. It is more difficult to relax under the influence of a stimulant drug. When people cut down on caffeine consumption or eliminate it completely, the results are striking. They frequently feel less stressed. They learn to identify when they are really tired and need to rest or relax. Moreover, they can relax more easily without needing a drink.

Both caffeine and alcohol can be pleasurable and useful drugs, but they are both physically addictive. We can be energized or relaxed without them and experience a quicker return to a natural state of being.

Loneliness and social isolation can be stressful. While many people need to spend time alone in order to relax or get in touch with their inner resources, most people need and enjoy a network of supportive friends and family. Working too hard, being too competitive, or moving too frequently makes it hard to maintain a circle of close friends. Recent research indicates that people with close-knit ties to family, friends, and religious, or other social groups have lower mortality rates from all diseases than people who are socially isolated. It has been postulated in this regard that one reason women live longer than men may be related to their greater interest in social and family ties. Men and women who have the personality pattern that has been connected with heart attacks – competitive, hurried, impatient, and striving – may be more vulnerable because they cannot make good connections with other people.

Overwork is another common cause of excess tension. It is clear that hard work is necessary for survival, especially in times of economic difficulty. Change and technological progress make it hard to keep up in any field without constant efforts to learn new things and alter our belief systems. However, each person must assess whether he or she is taking on so much that constant feelings of rushing or incompleteness result. If there is literally no time to relax, eat an unhurried meal, or talk with friends in your day, your life plan may need reassessment. Quakers consider it important to limit one's work life to have enough time for family, friends, and activities connected to their meetings. One well-known cancer specialist insists that his patients spend an hour a day doing something that involves play and fun. It's better not to wait until you're seriously ill to follow these prescriptions!

Inner tensions can be as destructive as those generated by the outside world. Anxiety, fear, grief, anger, self-blame, and a poor self-image are words describing complex and unpleasant feelings that assault us and cause distress. Counselling with a trained psychotherapist is often an effective approach to these problems. In addition, many people have found the consistent use of relaxation techniques very helpful.

RELAXATION TECHNIQUES

The goal of relaxation techniques is to enable people to calm down after periods of heightened activity. We understand intuitively that noise, conflict, anxiety, and hard work activate a part of our nervous system that is prepared for action in the struggle for survival. Another part of our nervous system functions when we feel peaceful, quietly aware, receptive, and relaxed. This part enables us to digest our food, sleep soundly, enjoy sexuality and obtain relief from muscular pain. Pulse rate and blood pressure decrease, and the immune system works more efficiently to prevent or overcome disease when we are relaxed. Many creative thoughts and important insights occur during times of quiet.

Relaxation exercises help in two ways. Firstly, they help us to return to a state of calm after episodes of anger, fear, or intense activity, instead of feeling residues of emotional turmoil all day, and, secondly, to maintain inner balance most of the time, even during great stress, by having a sure sense of oneself. This comes with time, practice, and self-knowledge.

Many methods of relaxation are helpful, and different ones are suitable for various needs and people. Meditation, silent prayer, yoga, biofeedback, using a relaxation tape, or lying quietly in a warm bath are all ways to relax. Herbert Benson, a professor of medicine at Harvard University, distilled the essence of meditation techniques from many cultures and religions into his prescription. Basically, it is this:

'Sit quietly and comfortably with your spine straight and your eyes closed. Breathe deeply. Silently say the word "one" in your mind as you breathe out. Focus your mind on your breathing and the word "one". When other thoughts come to you, let go of them. Develop a receptive and passive attitude. Do this for ten minutes, twice a day. As you turn off the outside world with its noise and pressures, and turn away from your own thought processes, your body will enter a state of relaxation that has remarkable restorative effects.'

Many problems of middle age, including fear of ageing and low self-esteem, are also helped by relaxation. Carolyn, aged 49, was a non-stop talker and a successful businesswoman. She came to my office because of abdominal pain, digestive problems, and tiredness. She drank a lot of black coffee to keep her going at work, and smoked cigarettes to stop overeating. She had written out a long list of physical symptoms that were troubling her, from headaches and back pain to cold feet. Almost none of her natural body functions were working smoothly. After listening to her problems and conducting a physical examination, I suggested that we try a brief relaxation exercise as a model for what she could do at home. Carolyn found it very difficult to keep her eyes closed and not to talk for five minutes. 'I couldn't wait to stop so I could tell you about another problem I have,' she said. Then she laughed at herself and added, 'I guess that's a part of my problem, isn't it?' Carolyn reluctantly embarked on some changes in the way she

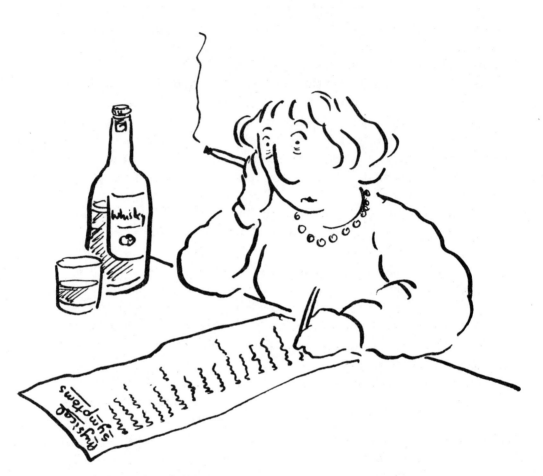

lived, including a twenty minute bath before dinner, with the
telephone unplugged, every night. In the year that followed she
tried several relaxation techniques, and found that biofeedback
worked best for her because she could measure her progress on
the machine. She ultimately bought an inexpensive biofeedback
machine to use at home. Most of her physical problems were
resolved without drugs, and she slowly cut down on coffee and
cigarettes. She learned to be silent without feeling anxious, which
made it easier for her to get along with other people.

14. EXERCISE IN MIDLIFE

Our bodies are magnificently designed to move. But after a lifetime of sitting – in schools, offices, cars, and homes – we often end up pain-ridden and diseased. Doctors are slowly coming to understand that many of the changes we have attributed to ageing are simply those that accompany physical inactivity. When young people stay in bed, they experience the same degenerative changes in heart and lungs, bones, muscles, body fat content, and digestive and nervous systems that we usually associate with growing old.

When middle-aged people exercise they can prevent, retard, or reverse many of these changes. The benefits of exercise include a reduced risk of heart disease and osteoporosis (brittle bones), easier weight control, improved appearance, decreased pain from many conditions, less depression, and better sleep. Let's examine these factors individually.

HEART DISEASE

Exercise helps prevent heart attacks. Though heart attacks are

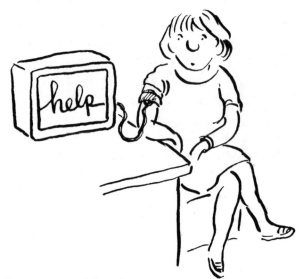

the leading cause of death among women over 50, it is not inevitable. The kind of heart disease we have seen in this century is relatively new – arteries blocked by deposits of waxy cholesterol have never been seen in such frequency before. Our overconsumption of rich animal food, smoking, and physical inactivity seem to be the culprits. In past centuries, heart disease was mainly due to rheumatic fever and other infectious diseases, or birth defects, many of which can now be prevented or surgically remedied. Yet the only lasting hope for the new heart disease – blood vessels plugged up with cholesterol – is a change in lifestyle. Surgery, like the bypass or replacement of blood vessels to the heart muscle, carries risk and only buys time. The vessels can become blocked again if the patient doesn't cut down on fat and start to exercise.

The combination of a low-fat, high-fibre diet and regular, vigorous exercise has a remarkable effect on the heart. Exercise makes the heart a more efficient pump, causing more blood circulation with each contraction and sending more oxygen to the muscles. As a result, you can do more without getting tired. This is what aerobic exercise is about. Any exercise is aerobic if it helps to condition the heart, lungs, and muscles to work more efficiently, consume more oxygen during activity, and so experience less fatigue. If you start a programme of brisk walking, for example, you may feel tired after one or two miles at first. But after a month of brisk walking, you will find you can walk four or five miles with ease. Your heart will have been trained to become a better pump. It will beat more strongly when you are resting, because it will be stronger and send out more blood with each beat. It will have developed new blood vessels within the heart muscle to nourish itself with oxygen. Your chances of developing serious heart disease will have decreased. Equally important for here and now, you will have developed more endurance and feel less fatigue throughout your daily activities. When you run for a bus, carry groceries upstairs, or dance, you will feel strong and capable rather than exhausted.

If you have exercised all your life, by all means continue daily during the menopause and beyond. If you have not exercised vigorously in the last month or two, begin with a walking programme. Work up to three miles daily of brisk uninterrupted walking in comfortable, flat, walking shoes. Walking is an excellent form of aerobic exercise which you can continue for life with great benefit. So is swimming or riding an exercise bicycle, a good alternative for wet weather. Before you start any exercise routine, check your general level of fitness with your doctor. This is especially important if you have any history of heart disease, diabetes, high blood pressure, or chest pain. A doctor's check-up is very important for middle-aged people who have been inactive and plan to start jogging, aerobic dance, or competitive sports. It is safer to begin with a walking programme and get conditioned gradually.

Dr Kenneth Cooper, an eminent cardiologist, recommends working up to walking two and a half miles in thirty-seven minutes, four times per week, or riding an exercise bicycle for twenty-five minutes, four times per week, with the controls (resistance) set so that a pulse rate of 150 is reached. He also advocates gradually building up an exercise routine including jogging, skipping, swimming, and other activities. Cooper's basic premise is that the heart becomes a more efficient muscular pump if you keep it trained. Just as our arm and leg muscles get stronger as we use them and weaker if we rest them, so does our heart muscle. A strong heart is a comforting companion in the second half of life.

But what about the waxy deposits of cholesterol in the blood vessels nourishing the heart? How does exercise prevent these vessels from becoming clogged? Firstly, it helps you burn calories rather than store them as fat. Secondly, it encourages the formation of a larger network of blood vessels to nourish the heart muscle, and in addition it makes the blood less likely to clot by increasing natural anti-clotting factors. Conversely, inactivity makes clotting more likely. This is another reason why heart attacks and strokes are less likely if you exercise regularly.

OSTEOPOROSIS

The brittle bone problem of middle-aged and elderly women is helped by exercise. This subject is thoroughly discussed in Chapter 7, and will be only briefly reviewed here. Bone fractures and back pain from compressed vertebrae are both results of progressive loss of calcium from the bones, which occurs in women after the menopause. Black women appear to be more or less immune from this condition, perhaps because of their stronger bone structures. About 25% of Asian, white, and brown-skinned women develop painful fractures from slight injury after the menopause. The most effective approach to osteoporosis is prevention, and exercise is one important factor. People who are inactive, or confined to their beds, quickly lose calcium from their bones. Conversely, people who use their limbs and muscles vigorously develop thicker, stronger bones. Middle-aged and elderly women need a daily walking programme for their lower bodies and some exercise for their arms, like a racket sport, gardening, modified pushups, or lifting three to five pound dumbbells (or heavier ones, depending on their strength).

All movement helps – the thing to avoid is too much sitting or lying down. People with desk jobs should wear walking shoes to and from work and walk some of the way whenever possible. Use the stairs instead of the lift for at least five floors. Do some walking during the lunch break. Jog on the spot or use an exercise bicycle at home, while listening to the radio or watching television. However you do it, incorporate vigorous movement into your day, every day.

Even sick people and patients in hospital should move around. Bones begin to lose calcium rapidly with staying in bed. Enlightened doctors prescribe leg exercises to their post-operative patients and encourage them to start walking as soon as possible. If you spend the day at home ill, remember to move as well as to sleep. Get up every few hours, stretch, walk, and work your muscles gently. Your recovery will be easier, and your bones will stay strong.

WEIGHT CONTROL

It's difficult to keep your weight in balance if you don't exercise. The small amount of food needed to sustain you in an inactive state keeps you chronically hungry and often undernourished. When small animals are kept in cages without an exercise wheel and given unlimited food, they tend to become obese. If they are given the opportunity to exercise along with unlimited food, they usually balance their intake with the energy output and maintain a normal weight. We function the same way. Weight loss is far easier if the dieter follows a daily routine of walking, swimming, dancing, or some other form of exercise.

During and after the menopause, women should not be too thin. The obsession with being slender in our society leads to great problems in self-image for most women at most ages. In the second half of life it is especially counterproductive, because thin women have less oestrogen and greater problems with hot flushes, vaginal soreness, and osteoporosis (see Chapters 4, 5, and 7). This is not to say that real obesity is helpful – it has definite health risks also. Find the middle way for yourself – a weight that feels good and can be maintained.

APPEARANCE

The person who exercises, using vigorous movement and stretching, keeps a look of vitality and suppleness in the second half of life. A stiff body is not an inevitable part of ageing. When middle-aged people start to exercise, amazing changes in their appearance are noticeable very quickly. A new grace comes from flexibility and energy. Yoga, dance, and Tai Chi are especially good forms of movement to impart youthful balance and grace throughout life.

DEPRESSION, MOODS, AND SLEEP

Exercise has subtle but extremely beneficial effects on our moods. The physical, muscular activity of vigorous movement stimulates the brain, causing the release of substances which produce euphoria or 'high' good feelings. Depression and physical pain are lessened. This is one reason why many joggers, dancers, or walkers get addicted to their activity. Some psychotherapists prescribe aerobic activity for depression and even go jogging with their patients. Any of us can experience a 'natural high' through movement. Many people find they are able to give up tranquillizers or antidepressant drugs when they begin daily exercise. They sleep more soundly at night, even in the menopausal years when sleep is often troubled by hot flushes. Anyone with insomnia should try daily exercise as one form of treatment.

Stretching exercises also help to counteract emotional problems. Tension is always accompanied by physical muscular contraction. Chronically contracted muscles are tight and often sore. As we learn to stretch and relax our muscles, our minds become calmer. The amazing benefits of yoga are related to this principle.

HOW TO START EXERCISING

The public has been exposed to lots of information about the benefits of exercise, and clearly it has made an impact. Joggers

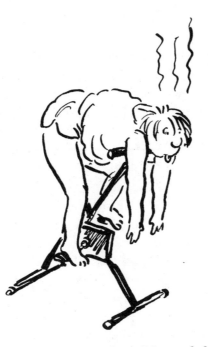

and aerobic dancers are all around us. Most adults, however, still lead fairly sedentary lives in our society, except for occasional weekend flings. The two most important realizations about exercise are firstly, you have to find activities that you really enjoy or you won't keep them up, and secondly, you have to plan exercise into every day, just as you plan meals, shopping, and going to work. If you don't consciously make time for exercise you probably won't get it, especially if you live in a city. Even people whose work involves activity, such as waitresses, farmers, or gym teachers, often do not get both stretching and conditioning exercises at their work.

Finding an exercise activity that you really enjoy takes some thought. Consider whether you want to take a class and be with people at a set time, or be by yourself working to your own schedule. Do you want to exercise inside or out, with music or without it? Do you enjoy team sports and competition, or do you want individual exercise with your own thoughts and your own agenda? Was there anything you did in childhood that would really be fun

121

to take up again, like swimming, skipping, cycling, or dancing?
Do you need different things on different days? Do you want to
join a gym and work out in your lunch hour or after work, then
have a sauna? Do you want to ride an exercise bike or use a rowing
machine while you watch the news? Go over the following list of
energetic exercise and stretching, and think about those that seem
right for you:

Energetic Activity
Vigorous walking, hiking
Jogging, race walking
Vigorous dance, jazzercise, aerobics
Bicycling
Using an exercise bike
Skipping
Racket sports
Energetic gardening or farm work
Cross-country skiing

Stretching
Dance
Yoga
Many floor exercises

Remember to start slowly with any exercise if you have been
inactive – patience and persistence really pay off. Above all, look
at exercise as a way to put fun into your day, because the right
kind for you will do just that.

15. DIET AND THE MENOPAUSE

Eating the right food is an extremely important part of staying healthy and feeling connected to the natural world. The optimum diet for the menopause and middle age is high in vegetables, whole grains, fruit, and foods high in calcium. Such a diet can supply plenty of nutrients without causing obesity or heart disease. One advantage of this healthy diet is that it is delicious, another that it is less expensive than a diet centred around meat and canned or packaged foods. When people change to a better diet, they often notice that many health problems slowly disappear. Energy increases, weight stabilizes, hair shines and stops falling out, skin looks better, gums stop bleeding, and constipation disappears. Let's look at the individual elements of a healthy diet and understand their pros and cons.

WHOLE GRAINS

Grains are delicious and can be cooked in many ways – whole as in brown rice, cracked or rolled as in oatmeal, or ground into wholegrain flours. The grain family includes wheat, rye, rice, oats, barley, corn, millet, buckwheat (kasha), and wild rice. Although grains have been a staple food for most of recorded human history, they have recently acquired the reputation of being high in calories. Perhaps this is because of what we put on them – butter, cheese, gravy, and mayonnaise! A slice of whole grain bread has about 90 calories, a cup of cooked brown rice about 200 calories. Asian people, who live on a rice-based diet, are mainly slim, in contrast to Westerners on a meat(fat)-based diet. The fibre in whole grains helps you eat more slowly and fill up naturally, so you don't overeat. In general, it is the fat in our food that makes us fat, not the grains, potatoes, and vegetables.

The medical advantages of whole grains are worth thinking about. Everyone is aware that something called fibre is good for you and relieves constipation. Fibre, the indigestible part of plant foods, is found in different forms in grains, beans, vegetables, and fruit. People who eat a diet high in fibre have a lower risk of contracting cancer of the colon, and also have fewer problems with many diseases of the stomach and intestines, such as diverticulitis, hiatus hernia, and appendicitis. They also have lower cholesterol levels in the blood, even after eating the same amount of cholesterol in their food. This decreases their risk of a heart attack.

It is also possible that a high-fibre, low-fat diet protects women against breast cancer. Women in Asia and Africa consume much less fat and three times more fibre than women in Britain and the United States do, and have a lower incidence of breast cancer. Many people add bran to their food in order to get more fibre. This is a good first step, but eating 100% whole grains makes more sense for your health. Bran is only one of the elements removed in making white flour or white rice. The germ of the wheat or rice kernel is the other part that is removed – it contains the B vitamins, vitamin E, and other nutrients.

Here are some guidelines for using whole grains. Buy or make your own whole grain bread without added white flour or white sugar. Use brown rice, rolled oats (not the instant kind), rye crackers, fresh corn, corn tortillas, polenta, and buckwheat (kasha).

124

Start the day with a whole grain cereal. Use wholewheat pasta, available at health food stores and now in many supermarkets. Gradually move away from white bread, cakes, and pastries to these healthier foods. If you like to bake desserts, use wholewheat pastry flour, which is entirely interchangeable with the white variety.

BEANS

Beans are an excellent food for several reasons. They are high in protein and low in fat. Any bean combined with any grain gives you protein of the same quality as meat, fish, eggs, or milk. For example, a serving of baked beans or split pea soup combined with rice, bread, or corn, gives you protein as complete as that in meat. Vegetarians are well aware of this, and often find they can easily maintain their desired weight.

Another advantage of beans is their high fibre content. The fibrous layer around a bean slows down its digestion, so the body absorbs its nutrients more slowly than those of other foods. Beans are considered the ideal food for people with diabetes because their slow regular absorption minimizes the need for insulin. If you are bothered by wind when you eat beans, soaking them overnight in water, discarding the soaking water and rinsing them thoroughly before cooking, will help. Fresh green beans and peas, beans sprouts, and soya bean foods like tofu rarely give you wind.

People who get much of their protein from beans and grains are helping the world food supply, as well as their own health. Sixteen pounds of grain and soya beans must be fed to beef cattle to produce one pound of meat. If more of us ate the grain and beans instead of the meat, huge amounts of agricultural land in the world could be planted with basic crops for the hungry. This fact has caused many people to examine their usual ways of eating.

VEGETABLES

Vegetables have always been pushed by nutritionists and mothers

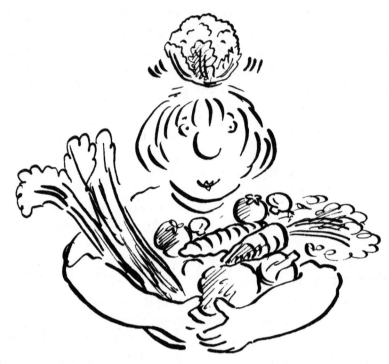

because of their abundance of vitamins and minerals. Now we are learning more specifically that they may protect against cancer, infections, heart attacks, and strokes. The evidence comes from recent studies showing that people with high intakes of vitamin A from vegetables (yellow, orange, dark green, and red vegetables) have lower rates of certain cancers. Conversely, it has been found that people deficient in vitamin A may be more susceptible to cancer and infection because of an impaired immune system. These findings should not inspire the public to take large quantities of vitamin A in fish liver oil or capsules, since this fat-soluble form of vitamin A can be toxic in amounts above 20,000 IU (International Units) daily. However, the water-soluble form of vitamin A found in deeply coloured vegetables and fruits is not toxic and can be eaten in large quantities. The vitamin C content of vegetables and fruits also plays a significant role in protection against disease, as do all the other abundant nutrients in these foods.

The information that some vegetables protect us against heart attacks and strokes comes from studies on garlic and onions, which show that they lower levels of blood cholesterol and decrease the tendency of the blood to clot. Similar effects are seen with root ginger and certain mushrooms.

To obtain maximum nutritional value from vegetables, they should be eaten raw in salads or lightly steamed. Water in which vegetables have been cooked should be kept and used as stock, because it is high in vitamins and minerals.

Sprouting is another way to obtain delicious food that is high in nutrients. As bean sprouts grow, their vitamin content increases. Anyone can make bean sprouts in the kitchen, from lentils, aduki beans, mung beans or many other beans and seeds. No other fresh crop is so easily obtained.

Potatoes and sweet potatoes are excellent foods which should not be avoided because of their alleged tendency to cause weight gain. They are not the problem – it is the oil and butter with which they are often prepared. Potatoes are best steamed or baked, and can be served with yogurt and chives or other seasonings. They are good sources of protein, vitamin C, and potassium, an important mineral for people with high blood pressure.

Sea vegetables are not used very much in Western cooking but are high in necessary trace minerals. With a little information, you can gather your own if you live on the coast – virtually all seaweed is edible. Easier still, you can buy small amounts of dried kelp and other sea vegetables at health food stores or Oriental grocers. Books on Japanese, Chinese and South-East Asian cooking give details on the use of sea vegetables.

As far as possible, avoid canned or pickled vegetables, as their salt content is unusually high. Frozen vegetables are a better alternative when fresh produce is not available. Don't forget to sprout your own from dried beans and seeds in the winter!

FRUITS

Fruits are an excellent source of vitamins and minerals. Use them for snacks and desserts, instead of cakes, ice cream, or biscuits.

When friends and colleagues bring out cake, sweets, or other sugary snacks, the conscientious eater can bring out fresh or dried fruit. For many people it is important to be supplied with healthy 'reward' foods if they are to turn down the 'treats' that lead to tooth decay and obesity.

It's true that fruits have a high sugar content, along with their vitamins and minerals. But their fibre content slows down the eating process and makes us full faster. In addition, the fibre of raw fruits has a stabilizing effect on blood sugar levels. If you eat two whole apples, your blood sugar will rise, just as it will if you drink the juice of those apples without the fibrous pulp. Two hours after the whole apple snack your blood sugar will be back to normal. However, two hours after the apple juice, your blood sugar will be significantly lower. This is because more insulin was released from your pancreas to help digest the quickly absorbed apple juice. The body responds to the juice alone in the same way it responds to simple sugar in soft drinks or desserts. The lowering of blood sugar after the initial rise makes many people feel relatively shaky, and soon hungry again. The lesson here is – enjoy the whole fruit. Don't make a regular habit of drinking fruit juices.

Some people don't like fruit, are allergic to it, or are on diets that restrict it. They can get all the nutrients of fruits in vegetables. Others wonder how to avoid the pesticides sprayed on produce. Wash fruits and vegetables carefully before eating them. When possible, find a market where you can get locally grown produce, and look for stores that sell unsprayed or organic products. These markets and farmers deserve our support. One advantage of local produce is that it has more nutrients because it is picked riper and stored only briefly. And finally, if you have a backyard or space for pot plants, start growing a few vegetables and fruits at home.

MEAT, POULTRY AND FISH

All are tasty additions to a healthy diet in middle age, but none should be centre stage. To have a low fat content in the diet, and thereby to decrease the risk of heart disease and cancers of the colon and breast, we should use meat as a flavouring for grains and vegetables rather than as the centrepiece of the meal. Oriental cooks do this by cutting up meat or fish and stir-frying it with onions, garlic, and vegetables. There are many other ways of changing to a low-fat, low-meat diet, such as making stews, casseroles, or soups using lean meat as a flavouring.

When cutting down on meat, it is not necessary to compensate with eggs and cheese. In fact, this defeats the purpose of achieving a lower fat content in the diet. Remember that a bean and a whole grain combination provides high quality protein without added fat. You can eliminate meat entirely and be healthy! Vegetarians have good health records, with lower rates of heart disease and cancer than meat eaters.

If you do like meat, how much is enough, and what kinds are best? Many heart specialists agree that middle-aged people should not eat more than four ounces of lean meat daily. Trim all visible fat from red meat and choose the leanest cuts. Discard the skin of poultry. Don't use gravy. The fat that occurs in fish is much less harmful than that in red meat, from the point of view of heart disease, but the oil added to canned fish should be drained. Avoid bacon, ham, luncheon meat, and pressed or processed meats – they are high in fat, salt, and chemicals.

Frying or grilling meat at high temperatures develops certain cancer-causing products. Use a lower temperature for a longer time, or cover the meat and let it stew gently in its juices.

Another reason to minimize flesh floods in midlife is that they may contribute to osteoporosis, or brittle bones (see Chapter 7). There is evidence that high-protein diets cause a loss of calcium from the body. Several studies have shown that vegetarians have less osteoporosis than meat eaters. To prevent osteoporosis, it is better to get more of your protein from low-fat milk products.

MILK, YOGURT AND CHEESE

Non-fat and low-fat milk products are good foods for midlife women because of their calcium content. Some adults lack the ability to digest milk sugar (lactose), and experience cramping, wind, and diarrhoea after drinking milk. Sometimes such people can eat small servings of cultured milk such as yogurt and buttermilk, where the milk sugar is partially digested already by the fermenting bacteria. Soya milk can be used as a high-calcium milk substitute.

Middle-aged people should avoid high-fat milk products such as butter, cream, ice-cream, and large amounts of whole milk. About 75% of the calories in hard cheeses of all kinds are fat – hard cheeses should only be used in small amounts for flavour. Low-fat cottage cheese, low-fat yogurt, and skimmed milk are good choices and also useful in cooking.

Many cultures do not use milk products and some Westerners avoid them because of digestive problems or dietary rules. Since calcium intake is so important in midlife women, those who avoid milk should eat plenty of the other high-calcium foods listed in the table on page 60 of Chapter 7, every day.

EGGS

Eggs are a high-protein food many people enjoy, and they are very useful in cooking. Because of the high cholesterol content of egg yolk, eggs have become controversial in recent years. Most cardiologists endorse the concept of a prudent diet where egg yolks are used in moderation – say three or four per week in middle age. It is much healthier to eat eggs poached, boiled, or baked in food rather than fried in fat. Cheese omelettes or soufflés are very high in fat and cholesterol and should generally be avoided. Powdered or dried eggs in various packaged foods should be avoided, as there is evidence that processed, dried cholesterol may do more damage to blood vessels than the cholesterol in fresh food.

People who are limiting their fat and cholesterol intake often use egg white and avoid egg yolks completely. Farmers who raise their own chickens and eat their own eggs should know that chickens fed only grains and plant foods have about 50% less cholesterol in their eggs than chicken fed meat meal, fish meal, and poultry by-products.

FATS

Butter, margarine, oil, mayonnaise, cream, and lard are very high in calories, yet low in essential nutrients. Those eating a typical Western diet consume about 40% of their calories in fat. This pattern of eating has been strongly linked to heart disease, strokes, and various cancers, especially cancer of the breast and colon. Recent evidence links a high-fat diet with high blood pressure, and change to a low-fat diet with rapid decrease in blood pressure. Since these diseases account for about half the deaths in this country, it is important for our society to change our eating patterns, moving toward a much lower fat diet. Individuals can do this without major disruption if they do it thoughtfully.

For health, we do not need to add any fat or oil to our foods. Enough fat is obtained from whole grains, vegetables, and lean or low-fat animal products to satisfy our needs and allow us to absorb fat-soluble vitamins. Most people, however, want to have some fat in their diets for taste and a feeling of being full. Therefore, the key concept is to use fat sparingly. Use just a *little* butter, peanut butter, or hard cheese in your sandwiches, with lots of salad. Use just a *little* oil in frying and avoid deep-fried foods. Make salad dressings with more lemon, vinegar, spices, and low-fat yogurt, and less oil or mayonnaise. Cut down by a third or more on the fat (butter, oil, egg yolk, and so on) required in recipes, and buy a low-fat cookbook.

For years nutritionists have advised the use of so-called polyunsaturated oils in cooking, such as safflower or corn oil, because these oils lower cholesterol levels in the blood. It has now been found that olive oil, which is a monounsaturated oil, is the most effective and healthful oil of all in preventing heart disease. Olive oil is delicious in salads and can also be used for baking or to saúte foods. Use it sparingly, and in good health! The only drawback of olive oil is that it is more expensive than other oils.

Eat seeds and nuts sparingly, and be aware of their high fat content. Be very cautious with coconut or avocado. Think of these high-fat foods as flavourings, not the centrepiece of your meal or snack. Fill up on whole grains, vegetables, fruits, and some low-fat animal foods.

Most sweets, pastries, and dessert foods are high in fat. Read the labels carefully on all packaged foods, and avoid those with added fat and artificial ingredients.

People who consciously change to a low-fat diet notice several pleasant differences. Many remark that they feel lighter, more energetic, and less sleepy after meals. They spend more time eating, and eat a greater amount of food, since low-fat foods are usually high in fibre and require more chewing. Yet they lose weight more easily and often stabilize at a weight considerably lower than before, without consciously dieting. Low-fat foods fill you up with fewer calories.

It's difficult, but not impossible, to find low-fat foods when you eat out. Much restaurant food is rich in butter, oil, cheese, and sauces. The conscientious eater can look for healthfood restaurants, and choose fish or chicken without added butter, salad or baked potatoes with dressing on the side, and similar simple dishes. When making air travel reservations, ask for a vegetarian or low-fat meal.

The recommendation to change to a low-fat diet is extremely important for staying well in the second half of life. It requires vigilance, but it is very rewarding in terms of one's energy and resistance to disease. It would be best to begin a low-fat diet in childhood, but middle age is not too late! The risk of heart disease increases after the menopause, and a very low-fat diet (plus exercise) is more important than ever.

SUGAR

Simple white sugar is added to cakes, biscuits, soft drinks, ice cream, sweets, breakfast cereals, and many other packaged foods. Honey, maple sugar, and molasses are added to many healthfood products. All these foods promote tooth decay and tooth loss, and represent substantial calories without nutrients. Sugar and syrups account for about 20% of our total calorie intake. When 40% of our calories come from fat and 20% from sugars, it's easy to see why many people in our society are overweight and prone to chronic illness.

For optimum health, eat sugary foods very sparingly, and satisfy sweet cravings with fresh and dried fruits. Many people do this by clearing all sugary foods out of their kitchens – from biscuits to ice cream and soft drinks. They find they cannot avoid eating these foods if they are in the house. If you crave sweets, stock your kitchen with fruit, including prunes, raisins, dried figs, and dates. Take some to work, and reward yourself for saying 'no' to morning snacks of cakes and biscuits. The sugar you get in fruit is supplemented by vitamins, abundant potassium, and other minerals which aid in its digestion and in many body processes. Fruit has fibre but no added fat or salt. People who eat fruit but avoid refined sugar have far less tooth decay and other diseases of civilization.

Many people feel really addicted to sweet foods, in the sense that they crave ice cream, biscuits, or chocolate daily and feel deprived without them. Usually these foods were associated with love and good times in childhood, and the association is hard to sever. It is best to work on this gradually, cutting down on sugary foods rather than cutting them out. Meanwhile, explore the beauty and bounty of whole natural foods and the exotic world of fruits. Focus on what you are gaining, not on what you are giving up. You will find it easier than you imagine once you start.

There is considerable controversy about saccharine as a sweetener. It has been associated with cancer of the bladder in some animal studies, but scientific experts disagree on the data. Many people use it extensively in soft drinks, coffee, and as a sweetener for desserts. In general, chemicals in food should be avoided. We already take in a considerable number of chemical substances from pesticides, herbicides, preservatives, and additives in food. It stands to reason that we should limit our intake of any chemical we don't need, especially if it is suspected of having adverse effects. In addition to avoiding saccharine, we should avoid artificial flavouring, colouring, and most other additives. Become a label reader and don't eat chemicals unless they are safe.

People who want a low-calorie alternative to soft diet drinks can drink mineral water mixed with a little fruit juice or a squeeze of a lemon. Delicious low-salt vegetable juices are also available. With enough consumer demand, more of these healthy alternatives may soon be found in supermarkets, cafeterias, and vending machines.

SALT

The sodium in table salt (sodium chloride), MSG (monosodium glutamate), and many packaged foods can contribute to high blood pressure and osteoporosis. Recent research has shown that the chloride part of sodium chloride may also raise blood pressure. For optimum health, most people should limit salt intake and instead flavour food with onions, garlic, lemon juice, herbs, and spices. The body does required sodium, but usually we get enough of this element in vegetables, fruits, grains, and animal foods. In societies where little or no salt is added to food, there is virtually no problem with high blood pressure. Conversely, in societies where food is highly salted, high blood pressure and strokes (a complication of high blood pressure) are very common. From the perspective of good health, most food in this country is oversalted. Not everyone develops severe blood problems, but certain groups are more susceptible to it. Genetics plays a part here – people with a family history of high blood pressure are more likely to develop the problem if they salt their food. People of Afro-Caribbean origin seem to be especially at risk of high blood pressure, and although this has been ascribed to increased stress from discrimination and pent-up rage, it may also be due to genetic susceptibility to salt intake.

Limiting salt means cooking with little or no added salt and using herbs and other flavourings instead. Although some convenience foods with minimum amounts of salt are now available in supermarkets and health food stores, it also means avoiding much processed food, like canned soup, canned vegetables, pickles, olives, salted nuts, potato crisps, tortilla chips, soy sauce, tamari, miso, and many packaged desserts. Any hard cheese should be used sparingly, because it is high in sodium as well as fat. Restaurant food is often overloaded with salt and monosodium glutamate, although some Oriental restaurants no longer use MSG (monosodium glutamate) or will omit it on request.

Clearly, it is difficult to be vigilant in this area. However, you can succeed in cutting down considerably and still enjoy food and life. In fact, a recent study of people who cut salt out of their diets because of high blood pressure revealed that they felt happier, less depressed, and less dependent on drugs, such as asprin, for pain relief.

Salt is an acquired taste. Children brought up without it grow into adults who don't crave it. And adults can condition themselves gradually to enjoy food without added salt.

The drug treatment of high blood pressure often has undesirable side effects, such as fatigue, dizziness, or decreased sex drive. There may also be unexpected long-term side effects to the powerful drugs now being used to combat hypertension. Though these drugs are necessary for some people, the medical profession is currently re-evaluating their use. Many people can successfully bring down blood pressure without drugs, by lowering their salt and fat intake, drinking very little alcohol, eating a diet high in vegetables, fruits, and calcium, exercising, and using relaxation techniques like yoga, meditation, and biofeedback.

Because of their high potassium content, fruits and vegetables are important in a diet to reduce blood pressure. Potassium is an element similar to sodium, essential to life, but having the opposite effect on hypertension. Diets high in potassium and low in sodium tend to bring blood pressure down. Potassium is abundant in beans of all kinds, potatoes, leafy greens, and many fruits. When steaming or boiling vegetables, use the cooking water later as stock in order to retain all the potassium and other nutrients it contains.

ALCOHOL

Alcohol can produce pleasure, relaxation, sleep, and relief from

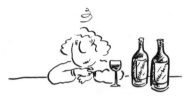

pain. It can also lead to disease and death. The effects depend on the amount used and the metabolism and personality of the user. The menopausal woman, and middle-aged people in general, should treat it as a recreational drug to be used with care and respect. Our bodies cannot take as much abuse when we are 50 as when we were 20 – hangovers last longer and feel worse! Let's examine the positive and negative effects of alcohol so we can make good decisions.

The positive aspects of alcohol for many people are that drinking enhances sociability, brings relaxation, and tastes and feels good. In addition, there is evidence that small amounts of alcohol increase a type of blood fat called HDL (high density lipoprotein) which protects against heart attacks, and that, in some societies moderate users of wine have a lower risk of heart disease. Studies of people who live to the age of 90 or 100 have shown that many of them drink alcohol, usually in a social context with family and friends.

Positive remarks about alcohol must always be balanced with a recognition that this drug has also brought terrible personal tragedy and social disruption to our society. Personality differences and biochemical individuality must explain why some people are addicted to heavy drinking, and why others feel toxic effects after small amounts.

There are several negative aspects of alcohol use in the menopause and beyond. Alcohol may act as a trigger for hot flushes. Heavy alcohol use has been associated with osteoporosis and fractures in older women for several reasons. Alcoholics often eat less calcium-rich food and excrete more calcium in their urine. They often have elevated levels of adrenal hormones, which act to break down bone. They exercise less, and have more tendency to fall. The menopause may also be more troublesome because of the toxic effects of alcohol on the ovaries. In general, middle-aged women who have used large amounts of alcohol feel much better when they stop drinking. Nutrition improves when the empty calories of alcohol are replaced by healthy foods high in essential nutrients. Often many other health problems clear up, like excessive fatigue, joint and muscle pains, or hair, skin, and gum problems.

Several recent studies from the United States and Europe have shown an association between alcohol use and breast cancer. Relatively small amounts of alcohol, amounting to three drinks a week, were found to increase the risk of breast cancer by about 50%. A drink is defined as 5 ounces of wine, 12 ounces of beer, or an ounce of hard liquor. The increased risk was found to be stronger among women who were younger, leaner, and pre-menopausal, and was found regardless of whether or not the woman had other risk factors for breast cancer such as a family history of the disease or a late first birth. The conclusions drawn from these studies by the investigators at Harvard Medical School and the National Institutes of Health were that further research was needed to help clarify the possible mechanisms by which alcohol exerts this effect on the breasts. In the meantime, 'the possibility that alcohol increases the risk of breast cancer should be considered in decisions about the use of alcoholic beverages.' My advice to readers is to weigh these conclusions carefully and to consider switching to fruit juice and soda water on most occasions until more information is available.

Alcohol has been connected to high blood pressure when it is used in regular high doses. Anyone with a blood pressure problem would do well to drink only lightly, if at all. In addition, alcoholic beverages are made with many chemicals unknown to the consumer. These chemicals may cause allergies, heart problems, or other illnesses in susceptible people. This is another reason to use alcohol with caution.

On the whole, it is best to be very careful about drinking in middle age. Analyse your drinking habits, and think about alternatives. If you feel you *must* drink daily to relax, enjoy dinner, or go to sleep, consider exercise, relaxation training, or counselling instead. If alcohol gives you heart palpitations (brandy and red wine can do this), or makes you dizzy or hung over, avoid it! Your body can't recuperate as easily in middle age, and must be treated with respect. Finally, if you have a compulsion to drink heavily, or other problems with alcohol use, don't drink at all. Go to Alcoholics Anonymous instead.

CAFFEINE

Caffeine is a stimulant found in coffee, tea, chocolate, many soft drinks, and some medicines. It affects the body in numerous ways, and is another recreational drug to be treated with caution. Most adults in our society use caffeine daily and are addicted to some degree to its stimulant properties. If deprived of caffeine, they may suffer mild to severe withdrawal symptoms, including tiredness, headaches, irritability, and anxiety. These symptoms last from one to four days, and then vanish completely.

Many people enjoy the effects of caffeine, and like the taste of coffee or tea. Is this a safe drug in middle age? What are its pros and cons for the menopausal woman?

Caffeine is used because it decreases fatigue, and stimulates the mind and body to work faster. People think faster and often talk more under its influence. Caffeine enables people to concentrate harder and work longer at many mental and physical tasks, but meditation and states of relaxation are more difficult.

In high doses, however, caffeine can cause excessive tension and irritability. Users become edgy and uncomfortable, and overreact to stimuli. Their hearts beat faster and they may feel irregular extra beats. Blood pressure rises. Sleep is impaired, and a state of fatigue follows. This can make people use more caffeine and perpetuate the problem. All of these drug effects are more pronounced with ageing.

Caffeine stimulates the smooth muscle of the stomach and intestines, causing some people to have diarrhoea. Hence it should not be used at all by people with problems like inflammatory bowel disease (ulcerative colitis or Crohn's disease). Other people with chronic constipation use caffeine as a laxative. The same effect

138

can be obtained, however, with a high-fibre diet of whole grain, beans, vegetables, and added bran.

Coffee has been associated with a rise in blood cholesterol, and thus may be implicated in heart disease.

Menopausal women frequently say caffeinated beverages increase hot flushes. This may be because caffeine speeds up metabolism and thereby increases body temperature. If hot flushes are a problem, cutting down on caffeine can be very helpful.

Caffeine has been associated with the development of benign breast lumps in women. It appears to stimulate certain celluar growth in the breasts, giving rise to more lumpiness and breast pain before periods. When women with breast lumps give up caffeine, the problem often regresses remarkably after four to six months. No relationship to breast cancer has been detected.

Very heavy coffee drinking (over five cups daily) has been related to calcium loss in women. It is apparently one factor that can lead to osteoporosis, especially if added to other risk factors (see Chapter 7).

In the menopause and in the second half of life, it is good to be 'tuned in' to one's body. When you're tired, it is better to rest than to stimulate yourself artificially with a drug. Following the normal ebb and flow of your body's energy leads to a more peaceful and productive life.

For optimum health, it is best to cut down on caffeine consumption. Some people find they can easily do without it, and enjoy drinking herbal teas or cereal-based drinks that resemble coffee but are made from roasted grains. Some drink decaffeinated coffee – best made from beans from which the caffeine is extracted by a process using hot water rather than chemical solvents. Some use caffeine only when they really need the stimulation, rather than daily. If you use it, do so sparingly, and be aware of its effects on your system. Weak tea with milk is a safer stimulant than strong coffee. Remember that cutting out caffeine may lead initially to caffeine withdrawal symptoms if you are a regular user. You may experience headaches and irritability for a few days but after this you will feel well again, and you will be free of an addiction.

MAKING CHANGES IN YOUR DIET

At 45, Lois had two experiences that shook her severely. Her brother had a serious heart attack, and she was operated on for a ruptured appendix. While recovering in hospital Lois asked her doctor why she might have developed appendicitis. 'Many people link this problem with a diet low in fibre' her doctor answered. 'Appendicitis rarely occurs among people in Africa who eat large amounts of grains and vegetable foods.' Lois thought of her own perpetual dieting on cottage cheese, hardboiled eggs, and lean meats, with occasional binges on cakes, biscuits, or ice cream. She found out, while in the hospital, that her blood cholesterol was fairly high, which worried her because of her brother's heart attack. The doctor, who was young and very nutrition conscious, told her to bring her cholesterol level down to avoid the family pattern of heart disease. As she lay in bed, Lois realized she had to change her whole pattern of eating. She called a friend at work whom she had considered a health freak and learned about the benefits of unfamiliar things like wholewheat bread, rolled oats, and various types of beans. Ultimately she found it easier to lose weight with this diet than it had been with her hardboiled eggs and lean meat. A year later her blood cholesterol level had dropped to a healthy level, and Lois had become a health freak in her brother's eyes. She was trying to persuade him to try brown rice and salad instead of steak and chips. 'I'm not a rabbit,' he said. 'Better to be a healthy rabbit than have a second heart attack,' Lois answered.

Most people find it difficult to break the habits of a lifetime and everyone makes changes according to his or her own timetable. Most people do better when changes are gradual, and when they emphasize the positive rather than feeling deprived. Women who are anxious about gaining weight may have an especially hard time changing from a diet that emphasizes animal protein, as they have been led to believe that other foods will make them fat. A gradual transition to a more plant-based diet is the key, with attention to your individual likes and dislikes. For new ideas on your diet and recipes, try reading several of the many good vegetarian (or low meat) cookery books, now on the market.

16.
VITAMIN AND MINERAL SUPPLEMENTS

Gina had a cupboard full of vitamins, minerals, herbal diuretics, and glandular extracts. At one point she took over 20 pills a day for a few months and then she abandoned them all in disgust. 'I'm not sure what I'm doing or if I notice any difference,' she said. 'The whole thing is so confusing and expensive.' Gina was anxious because she had had a mastectomy for breast cancer and wanted to avoid a recurrence. Finally her daughter, who was a nurse, sorted out the cupboard and gave her a simpler regime. 'Mum, you should take one multivitamin with minerals in the morning, and two calcium pills at night. That's three pills a day, and I'm going to throw everything else away.' Gina groaned as she watched all her expensive pills go into the dustbin, but she thought her daughter was right. At least she understood now what to take when and why. She felt more secure taking the three pills than she had previously felt taking 20.

A health-conscious minority of the population takes vitamin and mineral supplements daily, with the view that their individual needs for certain nutrients may be larger than average, or their diets deficient. Others consider supplements unnecessary, too troublesome, or too expensive. Nutrition experts often decry the inaccurate claims made for supplements, their potential toxicity in high doses, and the false sense of security they may impart to people whose diets are haphazard. With these viewpoints in mind, here's a simple regimen of supplements suitable for women during and after the menopause.

CALCIUM

Calcium is a mineral of great importance to the middle-aged woman, especially if she elects not to use oestrogen replacement treatment. If a high-calcium diet and calcium supplements (500 mg daily) are begun around the age of 35, as well as during pregnancy and nursing, women will start the menopause with thicker, stronger bones. The decline in bone mass that occurs after the menopause (see Chapter 7) will be slower and may not reach the stage where fractures occur. At the time of the menopause or at the age of 50 (whichever comes first) women would do well to take 1000 mg of calcium daily as a supplement in addition to a diet emphasizing calcium-rich foods (see table on page 60). If possible, take the calcium supplements on an empty stomach and in divided doses, 500 mg in the morning and 500 mg at bedtime, to enhance absorption. Take calcium carbonate, gluconate or lactate, not bone meal or dolomite, which may be contaminated with lead.

A great variety of calcium tablets are currently sold in chemists and health food stores. Most containers list the amount of actual calcium in each tablet. For example, they state that these pills each contain 500 mg of calcium. Some brands, however, give the weight of calcium and its accompanying compound, such as calcium carbonate, calcium gluconate, or calcium lactate. In general, calcium carbonate is the best buy, as 1000 mg of calcium carbonate contains 400 mg of calcium, while 1000 mg of calcium lactate contains only 130 mg of calcium, and 1000 mg of calcium gluconate contains only 10 mg of calcium.

Vitamin D is also necessary for calcium absorption. It is formed

142

on our skins by sunlight and found in fortified milk products, fish liver oils, and many multivitamin preparations. About 400 IU (International Units) are needed daily, but much larger doses can be toxic and should be avoided. Women who do not use milk products should be especially careful to eat other calcium-rich foods and take calcium and vitamin D supplements.

People taking supplementary calcium sometimes worry about developing calcium deposits in their joints or internal organs. This very rare situation occurs when the parathyroid glands, which regulate calcium levels in the body, are overactive, or when too much vitamin D is ingested. It is not a result of taking calcium supplements, which are safe for the vast majority of people. Women with any serious chronic illness or kidney disease should check with their doctors about any supplements.

Kidney stones made of calcium deposits occasionally occur, causing pain and medical problems. However, these stones are not the result of increased calcium intake, except in rare cases. They can be the result of a diet too high in protein or salt and too low in fluids because the excess protein or salt intake causes a greater loss of calcium in the urine, as explained in Chapter 7. During World War II, when meat was very scarce in Britain and Europe, cases of kidney stones were rarely seen. After the war, when the diet changed to one rich in meat, kidney stones increased.

MULTIVITAMINS

Multivitamin and mineral pills are useful if the amounts of vitamins A and D are not too high – not over 15,000 IU (International Units) of A or 400 IU of D – and if the entire formula is carefully balanced. The advantage of taking such a formula is that you are sure of getting many of the essential nutrients you need daily, which your food may or may not supply. Individuals vary in their requirements for essential nutrients, and a vitamin/ mineral supplement in addition to a healthy diet may benefit some people whose needs for a particular nutrient are especially high. Considerable work has gone into determining the minimum

143

amount of vitamins and minerals needed to prevent deficiency disease. Nutrition researchers are now also looking at higher amounts that may optimize health, and at the variable needs of different people.

There are several disadvantages to taking a daily multivitamin/ mineral supplement which should be considered. They can be expensive, using money which could more effectively be spent on food and other basic needs. Some people get a false sense of security from supplements and then subsist on fast food and soft drinks. In so doing, they are overlooking their need for unrefined carbohydrates and fibre and ignoring the risks of a diet high in fats and sugars. Finally, some people take huge doses of many vitamins and supplements in a haphazard way, exposing themselves to the risks of toxicity.

I advise middle-aged women to take a balanced multivitamin mineral tablet daily containing 400 IU (International Units) of vitamin D. In addition, I suggest they eat a wide variety of vegetables, fruit, whole grains, and some low-fat animal foods.

In certain circumstances it is an especially good idea to take vitamin and mineral supplements. Catherine, for example, lived in a halfway house for alcoholics where the food was inexpensive and rather greasy. White bread, luncheon meat, canned vegetables, and instant mashed potatoes were the rule. She noticed that her hair was falling out easily, her nails broke, and her energy level was low. She rarely took the time to buy any extra food, but she did get a strong multivitamin and mineral pill which seemed to make a lot of difference to how she felt. 'This is crazy,' she said every day as she took her pill, 'existing on this terrible food and making it up with vitamins. But right now I have no choice.'

Others who would do well to take daily vitamin and mineral supplements are people on stringent weight control diets who often do not eat enough to give them the necessary nutrients, people who have lost their appetites owing to pain or emotional problems, and patients with chronic diarrhoea, alcohol abuse, recent surgery, wounds, burns, or other illnesses. Consult your doctor to help tailor supplements to your particular needs.

17.
GIVING UP SMOKING

Harriet had been a smoker for over 30 years. She was a brilliant woman, a rapid and creative thinker who had written several books, and who taught history at a university. Cigarettes were her constant companions while she read volumes of material, wrote, corrected students' work, suffered through faculty meetings, and held court at a local coffee house with fellow academics. She punctuated her thoughts with gestures of hand and cigarette. Close as she was to her cigarettes, Harriet knew they were having drastic effects on her health and stamina. Her doctor loaned her a book on the health consequences of smoking for women. Harriet understood that her early and difficult menopause might be related to smoking, as well as her shortness of breath and extreme tiredness. Harriet considered herself a hard-core case in terms of her addiction to tobacco, but she also knew that she was a strong and determined person in most other ways. She decided to go to a stop-smoking course in a country retreat where there were no cigarettes for sale.

The course was extremely difficult for Harriet, but she

appreciated the information, the medical tests, and the group support. By the last day she could walk a mile without stopping or coughing. Several people on the course decided to keep in touch when they returned home. They decided to call each other every day to talk about their progress and with S.O.S. calls if they were tempted to smoke. Harriet stayed off cigarettes although it was the hardest thing she had ever done.

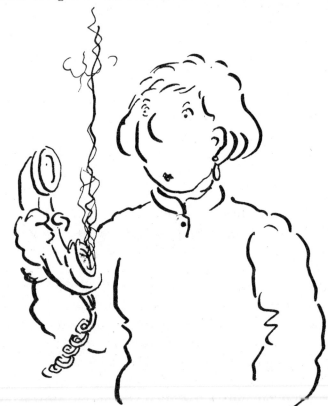

   Smoking has been mentioned many times in this book. Everyone knows that smoking is connected to cancer of the lungs and other organs, and leads to heart disease and breathing problems in the second half of life. It is less well known that smokers have an earlier menopause, and more problems with brittle bones due to calcium loss (see Chapter 7). Smoking is a difficult addiction to overcome, because it is tied in with so many aspects of the smoker's emotional life and daily routines. By midlife, most smokers have used cigarettes for 20 to 30 years. Yet it is possible to give up – millions of people do so every year. Benefits to your health occur from the first day of giving up, and mount over the years. Fifteen years after you stop, your risk of lung cancer is almost as low as someone who has never smoked. And, as far as menopausal symptoms are concerned, ex-smokers report a decrease in severity of hot flushes and a greater sense of well-being.

If you are a smoker, I strongly urge you to begin the task of stopping by becoming aware of each cigarette you smoke, and working out why you need it. Are you smoking out of a need for nicotine, out of habit or because of emotional needs not connected to a real craving for tobacco? Keep records of your findings. When you are ready, begin to think of yourself as a non-smoker, thereby tuning into the power of your mind and will to change your life. Get encouragement from non-smoking friends and loved ones, read a book about giving up, or take a course in it, and then throw away your cigarettes! Programme your mind to dislike smoke, dirty ashtrays, and cigarette ends. Stay away from other smokers for a while, until you are firm in your conviction that you are a non-smoker.

Many people who consider giving up cigarettes say something like, 'I know I should give up, but I just can't seem to do it.' Take a moment to analyse this statement. Using the word 'should' makes it seem that a higher authority is ordering you to do something, and you can frustrate that higher authority by refusing. Using the word 'can't' implies that there is an outside power preventing you from changing your behaviour. Actually, of course, it's all about inside you – the authority, the power, and the will to bring about a successful change.

18.
HEALTHCARE

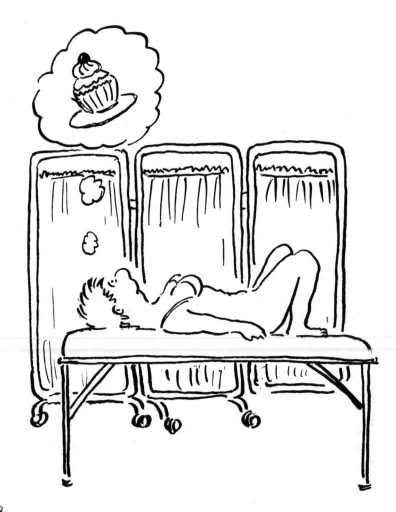

It is important to find a doctor with a positive attitude toward women, health, the menopause, and preventive medicine. You may choose only to see a general practitioner, or may decide to attend a special women's health clinic, as well. What is important is that the doctor you see is interested in women's health, takes the time to listen to your problems and questions, and performs a thorough yearly examination including a check on blood pressure, the heart and lungs, the breasts, the abdomen, the pelvic organs, and the rectum. Your doctor should teach you to examine your own breasts. She or he should also be able to advise you on questions concerning drugs, alcohol, smoking, exercise, nutrition and stress. A doctor with an open mind about the benefits and risks of hormone replacement therapy will enable women to choose what is best for them in this area.

Patients, for their part, should be as clear as possible about their problems, and should keep records of their symptoms. You should say when you want information, counselling, or nutritional advice. It is a good idea to write out your questions before an appointment, so you are sure to get them answered. Go to another doctor for a second opinion if you are worried about any treatment that is suggested to you.

Doctors who take a positive view of the menopause, and do not routinely view ill health and pain as inevitable parts of ageing, can help women with midlife problems. However, most medical education is disease oriented, therefore it is not surprising that many doctors continue to prescribe too many drugs for older women.

Bridget went to Dr Williams because of soreness with intercourse. She was nervous about the visit because she had not seen him in two years, and she feared he would pressure her to take drugs, as he did with most of his patients. Bridget was also anxious because she had just met a new man, five years after her divorce, and she wasn't sure how Dr Williams would react to her having an affair. She got undressed and waited for him to arrive while lying on the examining table. When he did a pelvic exam, Dr Williams remarked that she had a bad case of 'senile vaginal atrophy' and he pointed out the characteristics of the problem to a medical student who was working with him. Bridget felt angry and embarrassed by this episode. She accepted Dr William's prescription for oestrogen tablets in order to get out of his surgery as quickly as possible. Once home she cried, and decided she had to find another doctor.

She found out that a local women's health centre had opened a special service for midlife women. She went there the following week and had quite a different experience. She was given some interesting pamphlets on the menopause, sex, ageing, and the pros and cons of hormone replacement therapy. In a relaxed discussion with a doctor, she found out that she could use a small amount of oestrogen cream twice a week and not take pills for her problem of soreness. Above all, she found out that the physical examination did not have to be painful or embarrassing, but could be informative and reassuring. She came away feeling more self-confident and hopeful about her new love affair.

Instead of viewing low oestrogen levels as normal in the post-reproductive years, doctors may say that a woman's vaginal tissues are 'oestrogen starved', or showing signs of 'senile vaginitis'. Such attitudes on the part of the doctor can be much more painful than the vaginal problem itself. Hence, it is important for women to find doctors with positive views of the ageing process, which is why the newly forming network of menopause clinics in women's health centres is so valuable.

The same careful approach is needed in choosing a counsellor for emotional and psychological help. Midlife women should look for a well-trained person (such as a social worker, psychologist, or psychiatrist) with whom it is comfortable to talk. Look for someone who helps clients with emotional pain and encourages personal growth. Group therapy and midlife self-help groups are also available in some areas. This kind of counselling is more helpful for most people than the kind which routinely uses tranquillizers or antidepressants. As a rule, take as few drugs of any kind as possible, and make sure your doctor knows all the drugs you are taking.

19.
SUMMING IT
ALL UP!

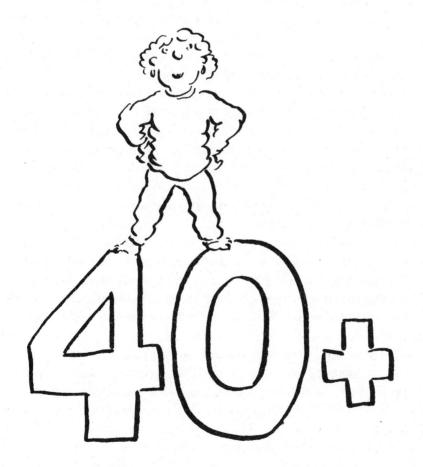

I have described numerous paths to the goal of post-menopausal zest, and have proposed a positive view of ourselves in midlife. Staying connected to the world, relaxation, exercise, a healthy diet, vitamin and mineral supplements, not smoking, and finding good health care are an important part of everyday life.

In and after the menopausal years, women have certain special needs, problems, and advantages. Their special needs are for more calcium, more exercise, and more attention to healthy, balanced living. Their special problems are those of hot flushes, brittle bones, and vaginal soreness with intercourse. Their special advantages are that the period of life after the menopause is smoother – no more premenstrual tension, hormonal mood swings, pelvic aching, or menstrual problems. No more concerns about birth control. Daily life seems to many women to have more balance and steadiness. Post-menopausal zest can become a reality!

In China, the sixtieth birthday is considered a momentous event, a time when the family gathers to celebrate the status and wisdom of the elder. Other societies which revere age have special positions for older women which acknowledge their worth and power. Ageing is seen as a gain in wisdom and not just a loss of youth. Interestingly enough, in these societies, the menopause is not viewed as a negative event, but as a time when women rise in social status and enjoy more privileges.

Can this be so in our society? Yes, if we make it so. Although our culture has glorified youth, especially in women, this emphasis is changing. As birthrates stay low and the life span increases we find an increasing proportion of our citizens in middle- and old-age groups. Midlife and older people are becoming a stronger social and political force. Two other factors are also at work – the sense of self-fulfilment and the women's movement.

The importance of self-fulfilment is growing in our culture. It holds that each person is not only equal but unique, and should develop her or his potential to the full, regardless of age, sex, or ethnic group. We can go back to college in our fifties, take up new interests in our sixties, change our names or our sexual orientation. This view of life allows midlife women to free themselves from the old stereotypes and gain a sense of self-worth. The women's movement does the same thing, and encourages women to use their conviction of equality and power in the world around them – at work, at home, in their local communities and in the country as a whole. Once women achieve feelings of real self-worth, regardless of age or appearance, they will not see middle age or the menopause as a tragedy, but as a time of accumulated wisdom and experience. They can see the second half of life building on the first half and developing from it in new ways.

I have discussed the special needs and problems of midlife in some detail. But what *you* do with post-menopausal zest is the next chapter – for you to write for yourself. Some women need to concentrate on survival or sanity in this difficult world. Others want to develop themselves in new ways they have not yet explored. Some women will become strong figures in their families, while others will be more active in their communities once family responsibilities decrease.

Do you need a model? Notice now many of the Nobel Prizes for Peace have gone to women – Alva Myrdal of Sweden for her work on disarmament, Mother Theresa of Calcutta for her work with the poor, Mairead Corrigan and Betty Williams of Northern Ireland for their work to stop the fighting in their country. All these women have used the special wisdom and experience of being female to inspire their action in the world.

One of my patients, Mary, spoke of her midlife changes very emphatically. 'I began to know myself in a new way after the children left home and I turned 50. I saw that my life was limited and yet unlimited at the same time. Limited in that I wouldn't live forever. Unlimited in that I could really be myself for the first time in many years. I decided to put my energies into local politics, which had always interested me. I feel I can use all my talents in working with and for people through politics. I'd like to see a lot more women, especially older women, getting involved in community leadership. They've got lots of wisdom to share.'

USEFUL ADDRESSES

FAMILY PLANNING AND WELL WOMEN CLINICS

Many areas now have a family planning clinic or a well women clinic, where advice and treatment for menopausal problems can be obtained. For your nearest clinic, look in your local telephone directory.

MENOPAUSE CLINICS

Some hospitals have a menopause clinic attached to them, offering both advice and treatment. You must be referred by your doctor to such a clinic.

ADVISORY SERVICES

UK

Amarant Trust
14 Lord North Street
London SW1P 3LD

Association of Sexual and Marital Therapists
PO Box 62
Sheffield S10 3TS

British Association for Counselling
37a Sheep Street
Rubgy, Warwickshire CV21 3BX
0788 78328
Useful source of nationwide information about clinics which provide counselling.

Endometriosis Society
65 Holmdene Avenue
Herne Hill
London SE24 9LD

The Family Planning Association
27-35 Mortimer Street
London W1N 7RJ
071 636 7866
Gives advice on all aspects of family planning, sexual problems, etc.
A good source of information about other clinics and services
available throughout the United Kingdom. They have a bookshop
and also free leaflets on many topics.

The Health Education Authority
Hamilton House
Mabledon Place
London WC1H 9TX
071 631 0930

Hysterectomy Support Group
11 Henryson Road
London SE4 1HL

Institute of Complementary Medicine
21 Portland Place
London W1N 3AF
071 636 9543

National Osteoporosis Society
Barton Meade House
PO Box 10
Radstock
Bath BA3 8YB
0761 32472

Relate (formerly National Marriage Guidance Council)
Head Office
Herbert Gray College
Little Church Street
Rubgy, Warwickshire CV21 3AP
0788 73241
Nationwide network of clinics providing psychosexual and marriage
guidance counselling. Local branches can be found in telephone
directories.

Relaxation for Living
29 Burwood Park Road
Walton-on-Thames
Surrey KT12 5LH

Scottish Health Education Group
Woodburn House
Canaan Lane
Edinburgh EH10 4SG
031 447 8044
Similar to Relate.

Scottish Marriage Guidance Council
26 Frederick Street
Edinburgh EH2 2JR
031 225 5006
Similar to Relate.

Women's Health Concern
17 Earl's Terrace
London W8
071 602 6669

Women's Health and Reproduction Rights Centre
52-54 Featherstone Street
London EC1Y 8RT
071 251 6580

The Women's National Cancer Control Campaign
1 South Audley Street
London W1Y 5D
071 499 7532/4

EIRE

Irish Family Planning Clinic
Cathal Brugha Street
Dublin 1
Dublin 727276/727363
Provides a similar service to the FPA within the confines of Irish law.

AUSTRALIA

Australian Federation of FPAs
Suite 603, 6th floor
Roden Cutler House
24 Campbell Street
Sydney
NSW 2000

Menopause clinics:

Queen Victoria Medical Centre
University of Melbourne
Clinical Sciences Block
c/o PO Box Royal Melbourne Hospital
Victoria 3050

Royal Hospital for Women
Paddington
Sydney
NSW

NEW ZEALAND

New Zealand FPA Inc.
PO Box 68200
214 Karangahape
Newton
Auckland

SOUTH AFRICA

FPA of South Africa
412 York House
46 Kerk Street
Johannesburg 2001

INDEX

acne, 49
additives, food, 133
adrenal glands, 28, 111
ageing, 47–51, 103–7
alcohol: 41, 111, 135–8; and breast
    cancer, 92, 137; and hot flushes, 34,
    35–6, 136; and menstrual bleeding,
    19–20, 21; and osteoporosis, 57–8,
    136
anaemia, 17
androgen cream, 45, 86
androgens, 27–30, 40–1, 45, 49
antidepressants, 69, 71, 120
anxiety, 65–72
appearance, 47–51, 120

back pain, 54
beans, 125
birth control, 43
bleeding, menstrual, 15–26, 100
blood transfusions, 23–4
bones, osteoporosis, 52–64, 77, 86–7,
    97, 118–19, 129
breast cancer, 77, 82, 91–2, 99, 137
breast lumps, benign, 139
brittle bones, 52–64, 77, 86–7, 97,
    118–19, 129

caffeine, 20–1, 34, 35–6, 62, 92, 111,
    138–9
calcium: in diet, 129–30; osteoporosis,
    52–64; supplements, 30, 59–60,
    142–3
cancer: 110; breast, 77, 82, 91–2,
    99, 137; cervical, 25; ovarian,
    28–30; uterine, 24, 80, 82–3, 86,
    87–8
Catapres, 36
cervix: 45; cancer, 25
cheese, 129–30
cholesterol, 90, 91, 116, 118, 127, 130,
    131
clonidine, 36
coffee, 20–1, 62, 111, 138–9
contraception, 43
counselling, 150

Depo-Provera, 84
depression, 65–72, 88–9, 106, 120
DES (diethylstilboestrol), 82

diet, 48, 50, 53, 59–62, 92, 123–39
dilatation and curettage (D and C),
    17–18, 24
doctors, visits to, 89, 100, 149–50

eggs, 130
emotional upsets, 18–19, 34, 65–72
'empty nest' syndrome, 67–8
exercise, 50, 52, 58–9, 115–21
exercises, Kegel's, 41–2, 43

fats, in diet, 131–2
fibre, 124, 125, 128
fibroids, 17, 21–4, 89, 99–100
fish, 128–9
flexibility, 50
fluoride, 63
flushes, 31–7, 84–5, 95
fractures, 53–5, 62, 86–7, 97, 118
fruit, 127–8

gall bladder disease, 88, 99
ginseng, 37
grains, 123–5
Gynovlar, 84

Harmogen, 81
headaches, 91
health care, 148–50
heart disease: 110; diet and, 126–7,
    131, 136; exercise and, 115–18;
    hormone replacement therapy and,
    83, 87, 90–1, 97–9; premature
    menopause, 77
herbal remedies, 37
high blood pressure, 82, 83, 90, 91,
    134–5, 137
hormone replacement therapy (HRT):
    78–92; advantages and
    disadvantages, 93–101; and
    emotional imbalance, 69–70, 72; for
    hot flushes, 36; and osteoporosis,
    62–3; and premature menopause,
    76–7
hormones: and emotional imbalance,
    65–6, 69–72; and hot flushes, 33, 35,
    36–7; imbalance, 17–18; and
    menstrual bleeding, 16; and
    osteoporosis, 62–3; ovaries, 27–30,
    41; premature menopause, 74, 75–6;

and sex appeal, 51; and weight gain, 47–8
hot flushes, 31–7, 84–5, 95
hyperplasia, 24–5
hysterectomy, 21–5, 27, 43–5

incontinence, urinary, 43, 87
infections, vaginal, 43
insomnia, 120
IUDs, 43

Kegel's exercises, 41–2, 43

laser surgery, 23
liver disease, 88
lubricants, 40, 86

mammography, 92
masturbation, 39
meat, 128–9
meditation, 113
menstrual bleeding, 15–26, 100
milk, 129–30
minerals, 50, 127, 141–4
Minovlar, 84
multivitamins, 60, 143–4
myomectomy, 22

noise, 110–11

oestradiol, 81
oestriol, 81
oestrogen: 27–8; creams, 40, 85–6, 96; effects on skin, 48–9; and emotional upsets, 69–70; hormone replacement therapy, 76–7, 78–92, 93–101; and hot flushes, 33, 35, 36–7; imbalance, 17; and menstrual bleeding, 16; and osteoporosis, 53, 62–3; premature menopause, 76; and weight gain, 47–8
oestrone, 81
orgasm, 44–5
osteoporosis, 52–64, 77, 86–7, 97, 118–19, 129
ovaries: cancer, 28–30; hormones, 27–30, 41; and menstrual bleeding, 16; premature menopause, 74, 75–6; removal, 23, 27, 28–30, 45, 75–7
overwork, 111–12
ovulation, 16, 17–18, 27–8, 51

periods, 15–26, 100
pheromones, 51
pituitary gland, 35
polyps, 24

potassium, 135
poultry, 128–9
pregnancy, 75
Premarin, 81
Premarin cream, 85–6
premature menopause, 73–7
progesterone: 27–8, 82; and emotional upsets, 69; imbalance, 17; and menstrual bleeding, 16; and weight gain, 47–8
progestogen: hormone replacement therapy, 80, 82–4, 85, 87–8, 90; and hot flushes, 36; and menstrual bleeding, 18, 25; and osteoporosis, 63; and weight gain, 48
prolactin, 74
protein, 60–1, 128–9
Provera, 36, 84

relaxation, 109–13
resectoscopes, 23

saccharine, 133
salt, 61–2, 134–5
sex, 38–45, 50–1
skin changes, 48–50
skin patches, oestrogen, 82
sleep, 120
smoking, 19, 21, 25, 33, 35, 49, 58, 145–7
spotting, 16, 17
sprouting beans, 127
stress, 18–19, 110–12
strokes, 91, 98–9, 118, 127, 134
sugar, 132–4
sunburn, 49
sweating, 31, 32, 34

tea, 20–1, 62, 111, 138–9
teeth, 54
temperature, hot flushes, 31–6
testosterone, 40
tests, for osteoporosis, 54–5
tranquillizers, 36, 41, 68, 69, 71–2, 81–2, 120

urethra, 43
urinary incontinence, 43, 87
uterus: cancer, 24, 80, 82–3, 86, 87–8; D and C, 17–18, 24; fibroids, 21–5, 89, 99–100; menstrual bleeding, 16; sexual role, 43–5

vagina: dryness, 39–41; infections, 43; Kegel's exercises, 41–2; soreness, 43, 85–6, 96

vegetables, 125–7
vitamins, 50, 60, 127, 141–2, 143–4
vitamin A, 50, 126, 143
vitamin B complex, 88
vitamin C, 126
vitamin D, 60, 142–3, 144
vitamin E, 37

walking, 117

weight control, 119
weight gain, 47–8
whole grains, 123–5
wrinkles, 49–87

yoga, 50, 120
yogurt, 129–30

zest, post-menopausal, 103–7